A Guide for Effective Clinical Instruction

Second Edition

Lynda Juall Carpenito, R.N., M.S.N.
Nursing Consultant
Mickleton, New Jersey

T. Audean Duespohl, R.N., M.S.N., M.Ed.
Director, Division of Nursing
Clarion University of Pennsylvania
Clarion, Pennsylvania

AN ASPEN PUBLICATION®
Aspen Systems Corporation

Alverno College
Library Media Center
Milwaukee, Wisconsin
1985

Rockville, Maryland
Royal Tunbridge Wells

Library of Congress Cataloging in Publication Data

Carpenito, Lynda Juall.
A guide for effective clinical instruction.

"An Aspen publication."
Includes bibliographies and index.
1. Nursing — Study and teaching. I. Duespohl, T. Audean. II. Title.
[DNLM: 1. Clinical Competence — nurses' instruction. 2. Education,
Nursing. WY 18 C294g]
RT71.C436   1985   610.73'07   84-21686
ISBN: 0-89443-573-6

Publisher: John R. Marozsan
Associate Publisher: Jack W. Knowles, Jr.
Editorial Director: N. Darlene Como
Executive Managing Editor: Margot G. Raphael
Managing Editor: M. Eileen Higgins
Editorial Services: Martha Sasser
Printing and Manufacturing: Denise Hass

Library of Congress Catalog Card Number: 84-21686
ISBN: 0-89443-573-6

Printed in the United States of America

1   2   3   4   5

To my parents, for their love
that gave me the freedom to become

L.J.C.

In memoriam to my mother,
Trenna A. Dahle, and my sister,
Dora Mae Douglass

T.A.D.

About the Authors

Lynda Juall Carpenito, R.N., M.S.N., is presently a consultant to educational programs and to health care facilities. Formerly, she was a clinical specialist in the nursing process at the Wilmington Medical Center, Wilmington, Delaware. She has held staff nurse positions and has taught in diploma, A.D., and baccalaureate nursing programs, most recently at the University of Delaware, Newark, Delaware.

Ms. Carpenito received her bachelor's degree from Seton Hall University in South Orange, New Jersey, and her master's degree from the University of Pennsylvania. In addition, she has pursued postgraduate study at the University of Pennsylvania. Duquesne University, and the University of Delaware.

Ms. Carpenito has written two other books: *Nursing Diagnosis/Application to Clinical Practice* (AJN Book of the Year) and *Handbook of Nursing Diagnoses*. She also authors a monthly column on Nursing Diagnosis in the *American Journal of Nursing*.

T. Audean Duespohl's experience in nursing education began at the diploma level and has continued to include teaching and administration in associate and baccalaureate degree programs in nursing. She was an associate professor of nursing education at Clarion University of Pennsylvania for twelve years and was awarded the Distinguished Faculty Award in May 1981. For nine of these years, she served as Chairperson of the Department of Nursing and was appointed Director of the Division of Nursing of Clarion University in 1982.

Promoting the use of nursing diagnoses as the basis for nursing practice is of great importance to Ms. Duespohl. She has been a member of the National Conference Group on Classification of Nursing Diagnosis since 1978, and was a member of the Task Force for 1980 until reorganization of the Group in the Spring of 1983.

Ms. Duespohl is editor of a book on issues and trends called *Nursing in Transition,* and an editorial advisor for *Nurse Educator*. She also serves as consultant for programs in nursing on curriculum development and spends a portion of her time travelling and presenting workshops on creative clinical instruction, assertiveness and nursing, and application of nursing diagnosis.

Table of Contents

Preface

This second edition, like the first is intended to provide concrete information for professional nurses in service and education who are responsible for the instruction and evaluation of others in a clinical setting. It will serve as a sourcebook on the mechanics of effective clinical planning, supervision, instruction, and evaluation. The book is based on two assumptions: that most graduate programs do not provide individuals with basic information on clinical instruction and that once given the fundamentals of clinical instruction, most professional nurses can provide excellent learning experiences for staff and students.

We believe that learning is a dynamic process that is continuous throughout the life. Thus, this book is meant to be used as a tool by the professional nurse in teaching others whether formally or informally. In order for instruction to be successful, certain fundamental principles must be internalized. Therefore, basic information is provided here for professional nurses who desire skill in the art of clinical instruction.

The second edition includes two new chapters, one on theoretical foundations of nursing education and the other on the relationship of creativity in nursing education.

Each of the book's eleven chapters concentrates on a specific aspect of clinical teaching. Chapter 1 provides the reader with a philosophical foundation for clinical teaching. Concepts of nursing, human nature, and health are discussed as the main components of the nursing model, and beliefs about each are described as they relate to the nursing model that is the basis of the book. Emphasis is placed upon the importance of teaching by a nursing model. Educators are encouraged to incorporate a nursing model into their curricula and nursing practice, rather than basing their clinical teaching upon the traditional medically oriented systems approach.

Chapter 2 focuses on the theoretical foundations of nursing education. Theoretical concepts include learning theories that have influenced the educational process and nursing theories that direct the practice of nursing. The teaching process is explored with emphasis on formulating objectives, identifying learner needs, establishing a learning environment, developing a teaching plan, and evaluating teaching effectiveness. These teaching principles provide a basis for clinical and classroom instruction and assist the educator in developing a method of teaching that is both creative and effective.

Accountability is the focus of Chapter 3, which traces the legal and ethical responsibilities of the professional nurse. Background is provided in order that one may understand the progression of nursing as an emerging profession and a practice discipline. The questions "Accountability for what?" and "Accountable to whom?" are answered. The client, student, and educator are shown to have rights that must be considered. Client and student rights are defined and related to the role of the professional nurse and nurse educator. The rights of the educator are also included in this chapter as they relate to the educational institution and the educational process.

Creativity is an important part of effective nursing care and nursing instruction. Chapter 4 details the role of creativity in administering quality nursing care and teaching nursing effectively, and stresses creativity in all aspects of nursing education. Characteristics of the creative instructor and of the student and the learning environment are described in appropriate detail. Blocks to creative thinking are identified and related to the teaching learning process. The chapter also deals with the fundamentals of clinical instruction and provides the reader with "how to" teaching strategies for teaching in the classroom and clinical settings.

An aspect of clinical instruction that tends to be underrated is the nurse educator's role in providing and promoting creative learning experiences. Thus, creative clinical instruction is the essence of Chapter 5. Clinical instruction is viewed as a nontraditional form of education in a nontraditional setting. Certain assumptions about nursing education and nursing students are explored, which provide a basis for effective and creative clinical instruction. Specific clinical strategies are identified for use by the nurse educator and examples of clinical focus sheets are provided to direct student learning. General creative strategies for teaching in the clinical area and their application during pre- and post-conferences are demonstrated for the reader.

The mechanics of clinical instruction are continued in Chapter 6 as the preparation for clinical instruction is discussed. The nurse educator in nursing education and nursing service is directed in techniques for planning and supervising instruction. The second edition has added guidelines for developing clinical focus objectives and more sample focus guidelines. Criteria for selecting and evaluating clinical facilities are discussed and outlined. Methods of assignment making are described and the advantages and disadvantages of each method discussed. The importance of clinical preparation for both the nurse educator and the learner is stressed, and practical applications of the teaching strategies are given.

Historically, nursing has been taught based upon a conceptual framework with a medical model as its foundation. In other words, the curriculum was developed according to body parts, systems, or diseases. Chapter 7 explains the use of a nursing model in clinical instruction, emphasizing the use of the nursing diagnosis and nursing care plans in nursing education. Nursing diagnosis is discussed at some length because of its importance to nursing education and nursing practice.

The second edition reflects additions to this chapter that represent the extensive developments in the area of nursing diagnosis and care planning. Specific strategies are presented for the teaching of each component of the nursing process and care planning in the clinical setting. The instructor is also provided guidelines for evaluating learner care plans.

Chapter 8 deals with communication and clinical instruction. It stresses the importance of communication skills to the profession and emphasizes the role of the professional nurse in counseling. Both verbal and nonverbal communication skills are discussed and then related, not only to the nurse-client interaction, but also to the teacher-student relationship. Practical applications of the communication techniques are included for use by the nurse educator in helping students of nursing to develop and perfect this skill that is essential for effective nursing.

Although Chapter 9 does not detail assertive behavior of the professional nurse, it does identify areas for its application. The nurse educator is advised to internalize assertiveness so that it may be used in professional practice and to use assertiveness techniques in dealing with students, clients, and other health professionals. Methods for incorporating assertiveness practices into clinical instruction are discussed at length, and practical methods are suggested. We firmly believe that assertiveness is a learnable trait that is essential for personal and professional autonomy.

Leadership skills are addressed in Chapter 10 with emphasis upon such aspects as change, conflict management, decision making, and delegation. The practical focus of this chapter is upon integrating a leadership experience for students into the clinical component. The nurse educator has a role as a leader in clinical instruction. Practical applications of the principles of leadership are described.

Chapter 11 focuses on the evaluation process as a vital component of clinical instruction. Evaluation is discussed as it relates to observation, recordkeeping, and behavioral competencies. This edition has given special attention to the dilemmas of clinical evaluation and specifically the unsatisfactory student. Guidelines for a grievance procedure and for counseling sessions are discussed. This chapter will serve as a guide to individuals held responsible for student and staff evaluation and will provide the evaluator with techniques and skills that should be used in evaluation.

After many frustrating hours as clinical nurse educators, we decided there had to be a better way to learn clinical instruction than by trial and error. We felt the need to include some simple techniques, shortcuts, and skills relating to clinical instruction that only years of experience in nursing education can usually provide. The teaching of students in the clinical area can be a rewarding, creative experience or a frustrating, debilitating one. We believe that the information provided in this book will aid the nurse educator in providing productive, humanistic experiences for students, and thus ensure the consumer of health care of a more dynamic, empathetic advocate—the professional nurse.

L.J.C.
T.A.D.

Acknowledgments

Our appreciation is extended to everyone whose continued assistance and support influenced this second edition. Our special thanks to:

- our husbands, Richard Carpenito and Terry Duespohl, for their cooperation and moral support,
- Olen Carpenito, for sharing his mother,
- all the nurses who have participated in our workshop and who have experimented with our ideas and challenged us,
- all the students throughout the year who have provided us with the opportunity to learn about clinical teaching, and
- our diligent typist, Maria Manel, for her thorough and rapid labor at the keys.

Chapter 1

A Nursing Model: Foundation for Clinical Instruction

Clinical teaching is the core of all nursing education. It therefore requires that the nurse educator not only utilize special skills and teaching strategies but also apply the conceptual framework of the nursing program to situations outside the traditional classroom setting. This demands that the nurse educator be proficient in the art of clinical instruction as well as able to relate the theoretical abstractions of the curriculum to the concrete realities of the discipline of nursing practice.

The unique strategies needed for clinical instruction are usually acquired by the clinical teacher through time, experience, and trial and error. A practical approach not only will enhance the educational experience of the nursing student but also will eliminate many of the frustrations encountered by new clinical teachers during the ''how-to'' period, allowing them to become creative and effective clinical teachers. Clinical teaching can be and should be learned through an educational process, not through trial and error.

In order to establish a frame of reference for the teaching skills covered by this text, a theoretical foundation will be outlined briefly. The application to clinical teaching of the theories taught in the curriculum is necessary in all clinical instruction and will be incorporated throughout this book.

Historically, most nursing programs used a medical model as the basis for instruction. That is, curriculum was based on pathophysiology and disease according to physiological systems. In contrast, a nursing model provides a theoretical basis for nursing related first and foremost to the patient, or client, as a person, not to the client's illness or disease.

Recently, nursing educators realized the importance of using a nursing model as the basis of their nursing programs, and they began to incorporate the emerging patterns of nursing theory into their curricula. In support of these new trends the strategies of clinical instruction are discussed in this book within the framework of a nursing model.

NURSING

Nursing has taken a giant leap from the days of intuitive care to the highly sophisticated care provided by professional practitioners of nursing in the 1980s. Definitions of nursing now focus on the client's individuality and active participation in promoting and restoring his or her own health. Nursing as a holistic and humanistic discipline is concerned with the care of individuals who desire assistance with health restoration or maintenance. Nursing is a therapeutic process involving the mutual interaction of the nurse, the client, and the client's family, collaborating for the achievement of maximum health potential. This process involves the sharing of health goals, pertinent knowledge, and available resources for the purposes of promoting health and establishing greatest well-being for the client.

As a practice discipline, professional nursing is provided by the nurse who has been educated to function in a leadership role within the health care delivery system. Focusing on the client, the professional nurse collaborates, coordinates, and consults with the client and other members of the health team to promote and maintain health. The professional nurse utilizes nursing diagnosis as the basis for all nursing intervention, and effects change through client advocacy, health education, health team coordination, and nursing leadership. The practitioner of professional nursing is directly responsible and accountable to the client, family, and community for providing quality nursing care.

Nursing education provides a theoretical foundation for the development of knowledge and skills necessary to assist individuals with their health care. Professional nursing education prepares the graduate to function as a generalist who utilizes critical thinking in the solution of problems reflecting increasing complexity. It promotes the application of the natural, social, and behavioral sciences, as well as nursing theory, to the practice of professional nursing. Through research, professional nursing education extends the knowledge base and scope of nursing practice.

Societal roles and trends interrelate with nursing and its survival as a service profession. The age of stress and affluence has directed health care toward the emotional and physical well-being of the individual outside of the hospital climate. Although most nursing practice takes place in the hospital, a great number of people who need or desire health care are neither hospitalized nor acutely ill. This change in societal needs has influenced nursing's view of the individual and family as consumers of health care.

PERSON

Health care consumers, known in the past as *patients,* no longer react passively to the health care system and its services. They have evolved from persons who submissively received medical and nursing care to persons who individually participate and collaborate actively in the planning and administration of all aspects of their own health care. It was this change in health care consumers and in nursing's view of them that fostered the substitution of the word *client* for the term *patient* to denote the recipient of health care services. The new term—*client*—to identify the health care consumer connotes an intellectually functioning person who has freedom of choice in selecting the health care best suited to individual needs.

The term *client* may refer to an individual or one of a group. It may identify a person needing assistance with health care or a family wishing to promote good health for its members. With this broad definition, the role of the nurse is expanded to include counseling of family members, supplying health information, and mobilizing the support system.

In order to understand the client better, the nurse must develop a basic philosophy of human nature under which to practice nursing. Although each person's view of the client will be different, for the purposes of this book we may make certain assumptions:

1. The client and his or her family are important members of the health care team.
2. The individual is a unified whole.
3. The individual continually interrelates with his or her environment.
4. Every individual has worth and dignity.
5. Given freedom of choice, people will make decisions according to individual priorities.
6. The person, as a sensing, thinking being, makes conscious choices and assumes total responsibility for the consequences.

The Client's Family as Health Team Members

For the purposes of the framework used in this book, the client's family is defined as any person or persons who serve as a support system for the client. This may describe a spouse, children, parents, friends, lovers—even pets. Whatever the composition, the family is a very important, but often neglected, component of the health care team. Its contributions to the well-being of the client are invaluable and must be considered when developing an effective health care plan.

Nursing has focused for so long on the client as one person that the concerns of the family were overlooked. Nurses must realize that the health or illness of the client as a member of a family greatly affects the well-being of the family. When a client is placed on a low sodium diet after discharge from a health agency, the life style of the entire family is directly affected. Food is bought according to the amount of sodium content, and salt is eliminated or at least limited in the cooking of family meals. Suddenly the eating habits of the family have changed. The family needs adapt to a different way of living because of the health care requirements of one member.

Since the family is greatly affected by the health or illness of one of its members, the entire unit must be consulted by the health care team. Collaboration with the family is essential if the nurse is to develop a realistic plan of care for the client. When the family understands the implications of the prescribed health care regimen, it can provide support to the ill member. A family's support of prescribed health care will promote client compliance with the established health care plan.

The Individual As a Unified Whole

For too long nursing divided the person into three parts: physiological, psychological, and sociological. Each part was dissected and investigated in an effort to meet the "total" needs of the individual. But by separating the needs into categories, nursing depersonalized the person. Categorization suggested falsely that physiological needs did not relate to psychological or sociological needs and vice versa. This led the nurse to view the client as "the gallbladder in 201" or "the schiz with paranoia." Nursing failed to identify the interrelationship of all human behavior and, in so doing, treated the individual as an assemblage of parts.

Eventually the emphasis in nursing changed to caring for the whole person. This notion must have meaning to each professional nurse in order for the concept of *total client care* to be internalized. When that concept is espoused without a personal commitment to its meaning, the client's rights are violated and nursing's responsibility to the client is denied. It is imperative that nursing subscribe to the concept of the person as a unified whole and that nurses internalize the meaning of that concept so as to use it in all aspects of their practice.

The Individual and the Environment

An ecological view of the person presents the individual as an interdependent, interacting organism who constantly interrelates with the environment. One cannot separate the individual from the environment, as each influences the other. Therefore, the person must strive to live in harmony with all the environmental elements in his or her life.

As nursing grows and develops a unique body of knowledge, it becomes more apparent that the main focus of the discipline should be the person. Consequently, nurse educators are seeking a more comprehensive and humanistic approach to the study of the person as a whole being. The wholeness of a person cannot be studied without the inclusion of the individual's life support system—the environment.

Realizing that both the person and the environment are dynamic processes is essential to professional nursing practice. The nurse must keep abreast of ecological factors influencing society and societal trends that affect the environment. Through this effort, the nurse will be better able to understand the relationship between the changing environment and health care needs.

Individual Worth and Dignity

It may seem unnecessary to discuss the importance of *individual human worth and dignity* in a book devoted to the caring and service-oriented profession of nursing. Yet nurses often forget the real meaning of those words in their efforts to get their work done quickly or to make things run smoothly. How many nurses have violated the privacy of individual clients during a bath for the sake of expediency? How many nurses have called elderly clients by their first names as a matter of course? How many nurses have argued with clients' family members about visiting hours? And how many nurses have then become irate because the clients responded aggressively to loneliness and fear? A nurse must remember that all individuals have worth and dignity and should treat them accordingly.

Freedom of Choice

Nurses and physicians have been making decisions for people under their care since the beginning of their respective professions. The medical information held sacred and secret for years by nurses and physicians made it virtually impossible for clients to make intelligent decisions about their own health care. In the wake of the consumer advocacy movement of recent times, however, health information is being disseminated by television, radio, newspapers, and other publications, so that the public is better informed than it has ever been. The American Nurses' Association (ANA), the Joint Commission on Accreditation of Hospitals (JCAH), and the American Medical Association (AMA) have made a stand in support of the clients' right to be completely informed about their respective diagnoses, treatment, medications, and health care. Information must be provided to clients in order for them to be active participants in their own health care.

The health team has long functioned under the guise of experts who know what is best for the client. Many times the health team inadvertently forces health care upon individuals who do not desire it. Physicians and nurses must provide opportunities for clients to make intelligent decisions about their health care according to their own priorities and not those deemed important by the health care professionals. The responsibility of the health team during the health care planning process is to provide information and suggest alternatives that will assist the client to make the necessary decisions. Clients must be given freedom to make choices based on their individual priorities and encouraged to participate actively in the planning of health care goals and nursing interventions.

Conscious Choices and Consequences

Decisions made by an individual who is acknowledged to be of sound mind and capable of making competent decisions should be respected by the nursing and medical staff regardless of whether the staff agrees with the decisions. This does not eliminate nursing accountability in the client-nurse interaction. The nurse must inform the client of the options from which to choose in making the decision and provide knowledge of the consequences of each choice. The client can then assume total responsibility for the decision and the consequences.

HEALTH

Health as defined by the client is the primary focus of all nursing. It is a dynamic, ever-changing state based on the individual client's ability to maintain his or her optimum level of wellness. A client's concept of health is derived from patterns based on age, sex, cultural experiences, and economic and other factors. Certain basic assumptions should be made concerning health and well-being:

1. Health is the expression of one's optimum level of well-being.
2. The individual is an expert on his or her own health.
3. The individual must be responsible for personal health care to achieve a state of well-being.

Health: The Optimum Level of Well-Being

The optimum state of health is perceived differently by each individual. For the young teenager, health means being free of disease and injury. For the professional football player, health includes pain and injury, which are part of the game. For the elderly person, health might mean being free of injury but not illness and disease, if one has a chronic disorder. Thus, one views one's own optimum state of health according to one's pattern of living. The client with rheumatoid arthritis may define optimum well-being as accomplishing the activities of daily living with moderate amounts of pain, whereas a client with COPD (chronic obstructive pulmonary disease) may perceive optimum health as successfully walking up a flight of steps without being totally incapacitated. Health is a personal experience that can be judged only by the individual involved. Health professionals must rely upon the clients to determine their own optimum well-being and assist them each in making choices related to restoring and maintaining the identified level of health.

The Individual As Expert

The individual knows himself or herself better and more intimately than anyone else. One knows if one is functioning at peak or if something is different in bodily functioning. Often when elderly persons complain of a new problem, health professionals attribute it to "old age" or "arthritis," without a second thought. But old age and arthritis do not attack a person overnight. Clients of all ages know when something is not right with their bodies. Nurses need to listen to what clients are saying about their health care and remember that they are the experts on their own well-being.

This, however, does not negate the nurse's responsibility to the client for quality nursing care. Although the clients are experts on their own health, they are not experts in the area of health care. It is therefore the nurse's responsibility to serve as the clients' major resource for health care and health care information.

Individual Responsibility for Health Care

Individuals, as rational beings, must be responsible for their own health care to achieve a state of well-being that is right for each one. Thus clients must be consulted concerning their health goals and be encouraged to become active participants in planning their own health care. Nursing care must be a collaborative effort between the clients, clients' families, and nurses, if health restoration and health maintenance are to occur. As a participant in the health care process, clients each have a direct responsibility for self-direction and self-motivation.

SUMMARY

Clinical teaching based upon a nursing model may be a new experience for many nurses already involved in nursing education. The nurse educator's philosophy about nursing, the individual, and health will directly influence the quality and type of clinical instruction he or she will provide. Therefore the first step in learning how to teach in a clinical setting is to identify one's beliefs and values about these concepts and develop a personal framework for practicing nursing. Once this framework for practice has been established, the strategies of clinical teaching can be learned and applied in teaching situations. When you believe, practice, and teach the nursing model, you will have taken the first major step toward becoming an effective and creative clinical instructor.

Chapter 2

Theoretical Foundations of Nursing Instruction

If nursing is to survive as an autonomous profession, then nursing education must keep up with changing trends. Nursing education should seek to identify and clarify its identity in the whirlwind of confusion among health professionals and paraprofessionals. In an effort to do this, nurse educators have sought to incorporate the emerging patterns of learning and nursing theory into the curricula.

THEORETICAL CONCEPTS

If asked, most nurse educators would not or could not identify the learning and nursing theory from which they derive their educational practices. Many might even say that they subscribe to no specific learning or nursing theory but instead have developed their own philosophical base for teaching. In truth, most educators either consciously or unconsciously endorse a theory of learning and an existing theory of nursing. Thus, it is important to have a fundamental knowledge of the concepts and theories about learning and nursing because of the influence these concepts and philosophies have had and will continue to have upon educational trends.

Learning Theory

The many theories about learning can be broadly classified as mechanistic, structural, and psychoanalytic. The mechanistic theory is derived from two British philosophers, John Locke and David Hume, who sought to describe the process of learning as a passive experience. A major proponent of the mechanistic theory is B.F. Skinner, who classifies himself as a behaviorist. Skinner's theory revolves around the power of reinforcement and/or conditioning. The acceptance of this theory relies upon the assumption that an individual is a passive organism who is manipulated by his or her environment. In other words, the organism continually responds to the stimulation of the environment forming a behavioral pattern. This interaction between the response of the organism to the multitude of environmental stimuli is referred to as the stimuli-response or S-R pattern.[1]

The concept of learning according to the structural theorists is based on the works of the Frenchman Jacques Rousseau and the German philosopher Immanuel Kant. Structural theories have been approached from two different views, the organismic theories of Heinz Werner and the cognitive development theories of Jean Piaget. Werner, the lesser well known of the two structuralists, views development and learning as a total process occurring from the global to the specific and from the undifferentiated to the differentiated. An example of these concepts would be the progression of the child from random movements at birth to more precise and fine motor skills as the child develops. Werner calls this principle of development "orthogenetics." All important to Werner's theory is the total organism. His theory of learning is structural in that it incorporates all aspects of growth including physical, social, perceptual, and cognitive development. However, unlike other structuralists, Werner incorporates aesthetics into his organismic theory.[2]

The concept of learning according to the structuralist Jean Piaget includes cognitive, perceptual, and intellectual development. Piaget's theory emphasizes the ability of the individual to use all facets of knowledge to reason abstractly, think logically, and organize operations into a higher complexity. The term "operation" is central to Piaget's concept of development.[3] It can be defined as a mental routine that internalizes or transforms knowledge. Both Piaget and Werner support the belief that the organism makes active use of the total environment. The environment functions to enrich or limit learning rather than direct the individual's outcome behaviors.

The psychoanalytic theories of development are based on the work of Sigmund Freud. Freud's theory, which is much more recent than the mechanistic and structural theories, was derived from a study of abnormal behavior of the mentally ill. It was based on human instincts and drives related to hunger, aggression, and sex. Freud's theory deals with conflict resolution and the thoughts, feelings, and emotions related to the attainment of satisfaction.[4] Later psychoanalytic theorists expanded Freud's theory to include learning and socialization.

Although few of the seminal theories of learning are currently accepted in their pure form, enough of their conceptual frameworks have filtered down to influence today's theories. Nurse educators should review the theories of learning and seek to identify concepts to which they subscribe. By recognizing these concepts, they will have a more concrete and knowledgeable base for their teaching activities.

Nursing Theory

For years nursing has relied upon the medical profession for guidance and direction in the administration of health care to individuals. Both nursing and medicine focused on the patterns of disease and methods of treatment and therapy. Recently, nursing has established theoretical foundations that emphasize the whole person and focus on health and illness, not disease entities. This move has changed the view of the nurse from that of the physician's "handmaiden" or assistant to that of an independent and interdependent practitioner of nursing.

Nursing is evolving as a unique health profession different from the medical profession. Nursing's unique role and scope of responsibility are being identified by the nursing theorists in an effort to operationalize the scientific aspect of nursing into professional practice. In search for a theoretical base for nursing practice, many theorists have developed and defined concepts and models relevant to nursing. The four most widely recognized concepts are person, environment, health, and nursing. It is through the identification and testing of these concepts and their relationship to each other that the science of nursing will emerge.

King identifies four concepts that are unique to all nursing practice: social system, health, perception, and interpersonal relationships. The general theme of King's theory relates to the individual and his or her interaction with social systems. King views nursing as a human process that assists individuals to assume responsibility for their own health care.[5] This process includes the action, reaction, interaction, and transaction with the health care system.

Rogers identifies five assumptions that are relevant to the administration of nursing to the client. They include the concepts that (1) the individual is a unified whole who is more than and different from the sum of his or her parts; (2) the individual's life patterns and organizations are constantly exchanging energy and matter with the environment; (3) the individual's wholeness can be reflected by his or her rhythmic, dynamic, and self-regulatory life patterns; (4) the individual's life processes continue unidirectionally and are irreversible; and (5) the individual is a sensing, thinking being like no other. Rogers views her theory as a humanistic model that provides a basis for all nursing interventions.[6]

Johnson's theory of nursing is based on a behavioral foundation. Johnson includes in her theory concepts about nursing and nursing practice, the nurse's role as related to society's values, the individual and his or her behavior, behavioral system balance, change in the behavioral system, and the individual's behavioral subsystems. According to Johnson, nursing is concerned with the individual and his or her behavior as nurses assist the physician in a mutual mission of health care.[7]

Roy's adaptation model views the individual as coping with the changing environment by utilizing four adaptive modes: (1) physical needs, (2) self-concept, (3) role function, and (4) interdependence. Adaptation problems may develop along the health-illness continuum and result from inadequate response to meet need deficits and excesses.[8] The problems are the concern of the nurse as nursing's goals are to solve the problem and facilitate adaptation.

Orlando identifies the purpose of nursing as supplying help to a client in order for his or her needs to be met. The client may require direct help involving personal contact or indirect help such as referral to appropriate allied personnel or agencies. The nursing situation encompasses the behavior of the client, the reaction of the nurses, and nursing actions designed for the client's benefit. The interaction of these elements with each other is the nursing process.[9]

Levine views nursing as a human interaction in her theory of conservation principles of nursing. Her four conservation principles of energy, structural integrity, personal integrity, and social integrity attest to the nurse as a therapeutic agent focusing on the individual's ability to maintain his or her equilibrium.[10] These four principles direct nursing intervention in assisting the individual during a period of altered or disrupted health.

Orem's theory of nursing applies the major concepts of self-care to all aspects of health. Orem defines self-care as "the practice of activities that individuals personally initiate and perform on their own behalf in maintaining life, health and well-being."[11] Orem's theory of self-care is significant to nursing because it provides a foundation for nursing practice in health teaching and assisting the individual to achieve his or her optimal state of well-being.

From these brief summaries of the key concepts and models of seven major nursing theorists, commonalities can be identified in each as they relate to person, environment, health, and nursing. Most nursing theorists utilize the nursing process in the achievement of health goals as established by clients and their families. Professional nurses and nurse educators must develop their own framework for the professional practice of nursing. In doing so, they will ultimately become involved with the concepts and assumptions of the nursing theories that now exist in the field of nursing.

THE TEACHING PROCESS

Education is a dynamic activity that involves the teaching process. This process is a complex activity that is shared between two or more individuals and involves interaction of the participants with a mutual goal directed toward some type of behavioral change on the part of the learner. Within this context, learning is the acquisition of new knowledge and skills that requires both mental activity and behavioral change. It includes not only subject information but also attitudes, values, interests, and perceptions. Thus, when learning is discussed, one must realize that more than classroom and clinical knowledge is internalized by the student. The importance of the educator as a role model must be recognized as the student consciously or unconsciously acquires knowledge and skills that are not specifically "taught" by the instructor.

Students enter the educational system with experiences that direct their educational goals. Their intrinsic and extrinsic motives will affect how they perceive the cognitive process and their role in the learning experience. Educational goals must be evident and relevant to students to provide them with opportunities to be motivated and active learners. Thus, learning occurs most readily when the information shared is deemed valuable by the participants and is satisfying to their life goals.

Learning is a self-directed activity requiring motivation, desire, and effort by the learner. It is an active process and requires deliberate choosing by the participants. This choosing involves educator and learner interaction directed toward establishment of the educational goals of the student. It is through this combined effort that students learn self-direction and self-evaluation.

In viewing learning, one must consider the learner. In *Teaching and Learning in Schools of Nursing,* Heidgerken described the typical student of nursing in 1965 as "a young woman between the ages of 17 and 22 years of age."[12] This description of the typical nursing student in the mid-sixties does not apply to today's typical student. In fact there is no typical nursing student of the eighties. Presently in schools of nursing, the student population is made up of the following:

1. Individuals who have just graduated from high school (male and female)
2. Individuals who have returned to the educational scene after several years of absence (ages 20 to 55)
3. Individuals with health care experiences (Licensed Practical Nurses, Nursing Assistants, Home Health Aides, etc.)
4. Individuals with educational experiences outside of nursing (graduates from other educational programs, B.A., B.S., M.S., and M.A.)

This diverse group of students presents many challenges to the nurse educator who is striving to provide optimum learning to all students enrolled. The varying backgrounds of the students should be considered in organizing classroom and clinical experiences. It is often very difficult for the educator to provide the students with an educationally stimulating environment in which they can all learn with equal comfort and ease. Regardless of the seeming impossibility of this task, the educator should strive to meet the educational needs and levels of all students. Thus, the learner is the focal point of all instruction and the learner must be afforded the opportunity to be an active participant in the educational process. This philosophy directly affects the planning of educational experiences for the nursing student.

Teaching Principles

To relate the general educational process to clinical instruction, one must have a working knowledge of the framework for teaching and learning. Teaching is defined as an activity directed toward the acquisition of knowledge on the part of the learner. It is accomplished through the active sharing of ideas, thoughts, and knowledge by the instructor. It is the responsibility of the educator to actively facilitate learning through whatever actions and strategies are available.

Certain teaching principles must be noted in discussing the teaching-learning process. The educator should:

1. Formulate objectives.
2. Identify the learner's needs.
3. Establish a learning environment.
4. Develop a teaching plan.
5. Evaluate teaching effectiveness.

These principles provide a basis for classroom and clinical instruction and assist the educator in developing a method of teaching that is both creative and effective.

Formulate Objectives

Behavioral objectives establish a framework for teaching and learning and provide a direction for learning and a structure for evaluation. They are written in measurable terms so that outcome behaviors can be evaluated. Behavioral objectives that are clearly stated guide the teaching-learning experience in a systematic and deliberate manner. Such structure should not be construed to connote inflexibility. Flexibility is one of the keys to successful creative instruction and should be demonstrated in all aspects of classroom and clinical education. However, boundaries for behavior have to be established in order for planned learning to occur. General objectives provide the framework for learning experiences and are usually written as course and/or unit objectives.

Specific behavioral objectives are used for classroom and clinical learning experiences. These differ from general objectives in that they are more specific and address individualized learning needs. In writing specific behavioral objectives for nursing courses, the educator should relate the activity to the student and direct the student toward action. If such objectives direct teacher performance, they are considered teaching objectives.

Both learning objectives and teaching objectives have a purpose in nursing education. Learning objectives signify student behaviors while teaching objectives identify teacher activities for facilitating student learning. Thus, if student evaluation is needed, learning objectives should be written. On the other hand, if

Exhibit 2–1 Teaching Objectives and Learning Objectives

Educator	*Learner*
The educator will:	The learner will:
1. Discuss the relationship of oxygen to the client's energy level.	1. Describe the relationship of oxygen to the client's energy level.
2. Relate the importance of good nutrition to proper oxygen exchange.	2. Explain the importance of good nutrition to proper oxygen exchange.
3. Provide information on diagnostic tests related to oxygen exchange needs.	3. List the diagnostic tests related to oxygen exchange needs.
4. Plan a simulation on oxygen exchange needs.	4. View a simulation on oxygen exchange needs.
5. Develop a study guide on simulation.	5. Complete the study guide on simulation.

an educator wants to identify behaviors needed to teach the student, teaching objectives should be developed. Both teaching objectives and learning objectives should be written in measurable terms in order to evaluate achievement of the objectives. Exhibit 2–1 differentiates teaching objectives from learning objectives.

It is generally agreed that general and specific objectives contain at least three elements. These include (1) who is the learner, (2) what is the behavior, and (3) what is the content. A fourth element is often added that identifies the degree of competency desired to achieve success. This last item is often eliminated in writing objectives because it is often difficult to establish a standard of performance. Exhibit 2–2 shows the four elements and gives an example of each.

During the process of writing behavioral objectives for the learning experience, the educator must determine the domain and level of each learning activity. In *The Taxonomy of Educational Objectives,* Bloom et al. categorize three domains of instructional objectives: cognitive, affective, and psychomotor learning behaviors.[13]

Exhibit 2–2 Objective Elements

OBJECTIVE: The student will list four symptoms of altered oxygen exchange.

1. Who is the learner?	Nursing student
2. What behavior is expected?	List the items
3. What is the content?	Symptoms of altered oxygen exchange
4. What is the degree of competency?	Know four items

Cognitive behavior is intellectual and ranges from the learning of simple facts to the more complex activities of synthesis and evaluation. Cognitive learning includes knowledge, comprehension, application, analysis, synthesis, and evaluation. The lowest level of cognitive learning is knowledge where the individual memorizes facts and terms for recall at a later time. Comprehension is the next level of behavior and represents the first step to understanding. It is at this level that the learner is able to problem solve or provide explanations without full knowledge of content. The use of ideas, facts, and principles in a concrete situation describes the cognitive level of application. Analysis deals with the breaking down of knowledge into relevant parts. The next step, synthesis, involves the building up of a pattern or structure from individual elements or parts. The highest level in the cognitive domain is evaluation. During evaluation the learner must make judgments about predetermined criteria. Such decision making can be quantitative or qualitative about the value or the purpose of knowledge, solutions, materials, etc. Exhibit 2–3 presents behavioral objectives in each level of the cognitive domain.

The affective domain includes receiving, responding, valuing, organizing, and internalizing. Affective learning is the most difficult to evaluate because it involves individual feelings, attitudes, and values. Educators differ on the importance of writing behavioral objectives in this domain since it is so personal in nature. Fear of invasion of privacy is often the reason for nurse educators to eliminate this group from the behavioral objectives written for classroom and/or clinical learning.

The lowest level in the affective domain is receiving. In this behavior, the individual is aware of a situation but rarely invests emotional interest in the learning behavior. Responding is the next level of behavior and is demonstrated

---

Exhibit 2–3 Cognitive Domain and Objectives

Cognitive Domain	Objectives
1. Knowledge	1. The students will list three hazards of immobility.
2. Comprehension	2. The student will explain how immobility affects the circulatory system.
3. Application	3. The student will demonstrate the nursing interventions used to prevent decubiti on an immobile client in traction.
4. Analysis	4. The student will explain the relationship between the circulatory system and urinary system of an immobile client.
5. Synthesis	5. The student will organize a plan of care for an immobile client in traction.
6. Evaluation	6. The student will describe two nursing interventions that could be improved in caring for the immobile client in traction.

when the learner reacts to the situation. Feelings and emotions may or may not be part of the individual's behavior during this level of affective learning. During the next level, the learner analyzes the situation and makes value judgments about its worth. This level is a covert activity called valuing. The next level in the affective domain is also covert and is called organizing. Organizing begins a higher form of learning as the individual plans and organizes values and attitudes into a systematic pattern according to established priorities. The highest level in the affective domain is the internalizing of established values into a personal philosophy of life. After internalization, the learner functions according to the values, mores, attitudes, and beliefs that have been accepted and integrated into his or her personality. Exhibit 2–4 presents behavioral objectives in each level of the affective domain.

The psychomotor domain does not have one set of agreed upon levels of behavior. Dave lists five levels that relate to psychomotor skills which include imitation, manipulation, precision, articulation, and naturalization.[14] Tuckman identifies the following three major levels in this domain: integration, application, and acquisition.[15] Simpson lists the levels as perceptions, set, guided response, mechanism, complex overt response, adaptation, and origination.[16]

It can be seen by the three groupings that a taxonomy for this domain not only has not been agreed upon but is also not as refined as the ones for the cognitive and affective domains. However, similarities do exist. The lowest level of behavior in each deals with a thought process related to an action and/or an automatic act that involves minimal conscious effort. At the highest level the behavior of the learner integrates a pattern into his or her life that is routine and spontaneous.

Learning occurs in three domains, cognitive, affective, and psychomotor. Although each domain identifies independent behaviors, the three are interde-

---

Exhibit 2–4 Affective Domain and Objectives

Affective Domain	*Objectives*
1. Receiving	1. The student will recognize the importance of client input in developing a plan of care.
2. Responding	2. The student will interact with the client in developing a plan of care.
3. Valuing	3. The student will assume responsibility for collaborating with the client and family about client care.
4. Organizing	4. The student will develop a plan of care based on client and family input.
5. Internalizing	5. The student will integrate the concept that the client is an "expert" on his or her health into the plan of care.

pendent in their application to writing objectives. All three domains are relevant to nursing since nursing activities usually include a combination of all three types of behaviors at different levels. Appendix 2–A lists behavioral verbs that are appropriate for each level of the three taxonomies.

Behavioral objectives indicate the desired behavior that the learner is to achieve. When clearly written, behavioral objectives provide a mechanism for educators to evaluate learner performance. In addition, students have a method for determining their own progress in attaining the educational goals. Behavioral objectives written in nonbehavioral terms do not foster evaluation by the educator or the students. Thus in writing objectives, the educator should identify the desired behavior and write the objective accordingly. See Exhibit 2–5 for examples of good behavioral objectives.

Identify the Learner Needs

To some degree learner needs must be considered prior to the formulation of course objectives on a general basis and then again before the specific classroom content is developed. Knowing the needs of the students provides direction for the educator in developing a plan for teaching. However, after the formulation of program, level, course, and unit objectives, the instructor must again evaluate student learning needs. The educator should:

- Assess learning needs of students.
- Pretest students for incoming knowledge.
- Develop learning experiences based on results.
- Implement teaching strategies to meet learning needs.
- Post-test students for outcome knowledge.

Exhibit 2–5 Behavioral Objectives

Nonbehavioral	*Behavioral*
The student will:	The student will:
1. Know four safety hazards in the hospital.	1. List four safety hazards in the hospital.
2. Understand the relationships between oxygen and fire.	2. Identify factors that create safety hazards when oxygen is in use.
3. Believe that smoking is bad for one's health.	3. Describe the effects of smoking on the well-being of the client.
4. Grasp the importance of safety to one's well-being.	4. Explain the importance of safety to one's well-being.

In nursing education, students enter courses with a variety of knowledge and needs. The knowledge may be from previous experiences related to nursing or it may come from educational experiences in other academic disciplines. The diverse backgrounds of students mean that each has individual needs. The needs may be related to subject matter, study habits, rate of learning, self-direction, or personal learning habits. Individual students have unique learning needs. They differ in their motivation, interest, and attitudes toward learning. The educator should consider all these factors when developing a teaching plan.

The educator must develop teaching methods that meet the individual needs of the learners in the classroom and the clinical setting. The importance of teaching to the individualized needs of the learner cannot be overemphasized. As a class, individual needs often become lost in the group objectives. It is therefore imperative that the educator view the class as a group of individuals with separate as well as collective needs.

In the classroom, students should have the opportunity to determine their own educational goals. In establishing these goals, students are given the freedom to choose what is important and satisfying to them. From available opportunities, they can select those activities that would best meet their learning needs. In doing this, students assume responsibility for their own goals and the experiences that will assist them in accomplishing their objectives. In this type of environment the instructor would educate by facilitation. The educator would determine broad course content, and a joint student-teacher decision would identify meaningful educational experiences. While one student may choose to learn by reading, another may select to view films, videotapes, or filmstrips to master the content. Such teaching strategies permit the students to grow in decision making and allow them to assume responsibility for their choices.

Individualized teaching can also be applied to student learning experiences in the clinical setting. One method of meeting the individual needs of students might be to encourage them to design their own educational objectives related to the clinical objectives already established. This experience for students might take place in the community, such as public schools, organizations, homes, or in the traditional hospital setting. The choice of experiences could also be determined by the students and their individual learning needs. Joint planning between students and faculty allows students to be actively involved in the educational process and select those experiences and opportunities that will meet their individual needs.

Establish A Learning Environment

It is the responsibility of the nurse educator to provide an environment that is conducive to learning. A relaxed but professional climate will promote inquiry and discovery by students. In addition, the nurse educator should establish an atmosphere that provides freedom for learning, positive reinforcement, and an attitude of acceptance. An open environment fosters positive feelings in students in which they feel safe to succeed or fail. This type of educational environment will aid the student to internalize concepts and principles essential to the practice of nursing.

The personality of the nurse educator can also influence the learning that occurs by students. O'Shea and Parsons conducted a study involving 205 students and 24 faculty that sought to determine the relationship of faculty behaviors to student learning. The participants were asked two questions:

- What faculty behaviors facilitate learning in the clinical setting?
- What faculty behaviors interfere with learning in the clinical setting?

Personal attributes of the faculty identified as facilitators to learning were "supportive," "concerned," "understanding," and "friendly." Characteristics that were identified as inhibitors to learning were "authoritarian," "intimidating," "critical in the presence of others," and "impersonal."[17]

Rogers has identified three concepts that facilitate positive interactions and thus influence learning. These concepts are empathy, congruence, and positive regard.[18] Utilizing these concepts, Karns and Schwab asked 31 students to identify five behaviors that promote positive relationships between faculty and students. Ninety-three percent of the students listed the following empathetic behaviors as enhancing interpersonal relationships: "understanding," "sees students as individuals," "realistic expectations," "cares about students," "knows students," "sensitive to students' other problems," "willing to help," and "remembers that he/she was once a student." Under the characteristic of congruence, over 65 percent of the students identified the following: "shares self," "will admit mistakes," "willing to evaluate self as human," "acknowledges limitations," "can accept criticism," "can relate on person-to-person level," and "honest." Over 80 percent of the students described behaviors depicting the attribute of positive regard. These behaviors included "gives positive feedback," "trusts students," "respects students," "receptive to student input," "willing to listen to student," "acceptance," "promotes discussion and questioning," and "treats students as intelligent individuals." Two other categories not falling under Rogers' three concepts were the availability of the instructor—identified by over 51 percent—and the ability and/or knowledge base of the instructor—mentioned by over 25 percent.[19]

In order to examine oneself as a role model and facilitator of a positive learning environment, nurse educators should review their instructional practices. Exhibit 2–6 provides guidelines for educators to follow in evaluating their behaviors by using the concepts of empathy, congruence, and positive regard.

As a facilitator and director of learning, the educator serves as a role model who exemplifies all the attributes of a caring, compassionate, and competent professional nurse. The characteristics of caring and compassion are exhibited through

Exhibit 2–6 Evaluation of Educators' Behaviors

Empathy

- Are my expectations realistic regarding student preparation the night before clinical practice?
- Am I sensitive to students' other problems (ill child, need to work)?
- Would I like myself as a clinical instructor?

Congruence

- Do I share some of myself with my students?
- Do students see me as exclusively interested only in nursing?
- Do I share my mistakes and limitations with students?
- Do students see me as real and human or stiff and contrived?

Positive Regard

- Am I afraid to allow students to practice without direct supervision?
- How do I respond when students challenge me?
- How do I respond when students make an error?
- Do I criticize students in the presence of others?
- Do I treat students in the same manner as I do my professional colleagues?

---

all personal and professional interactions. Competency of the educator must be maintained by an educational regime that includes self-evaluation, peer review, student evaluation, and self-directed learning.

It is the responsibility of the nurse educator to provide an educationally stimulating environment in which students can learn. This is done through the establishment of an educational climate that not only provides for the individual learning of the students but also stimulates the students toward self-direction and self-actualization. In addition, the educator should exhibit attributes conducive to positive interactions with students. The combination of these will provide an environment for learning that will motivate students toward fulfillment of their highest potential.

Develop A Teaching Plan

Teaching plans identify those activities of the educator that are arranged to meet the course objectives. Such plans are rarely developed by nurse faculty, although they are used extensively for client teaching by clinical specialists. They provide a framework within which the educator can work in developing appropriate classroom and clinical experiences.

The teaching plan is a written outline of objectives, activities, instructional methods, and teaching aids that are to be used by the educator during a specific period of instruction. Since this takes time and thought, the resulting instructional session involves a conscious plan of action by the educator. It eliminates the haphazard teaching that often occurs when instructors have taught the same material over a lengthy period. This means that classroom and clinical learning experiences are organized and deliberate, and not an "off-the-cuff" group of activities provided by the educator who hopes that learning will take place.

Although the teaching plan is designed to establish a framework for learning, it should be flexible enough to allow for constructive variations. If students demonstrate interest in a particular aspect of the planned experience, it may be beneficial for the educator to alter activities in order to meet the needs of the learners. On the other hand, such diversions should not dominate the teaching plans of the educator; and every attempt should be made to cover all the activities listed.

Every classroom experience should be developed as a separate lesson plan. This will allow the educator to plan specific learning activities for the students. If more than one classroom experience is included in the teaching plan, the content of the plan becomes so broad that guidelines for action are general and vague. Exhibit 2–7 presents an example of a teaching plan format.

Writing a teaching plan provides the educator with a record of classroom and clinical activities. These plans can be reviewed and evaluated periodically to determine their effectiveness. The educator can revise the material on the plan to meet the learning needs of the students. In effect, the plans serve to document the learning experiences of students.

Evaluate Teaching Effectiveness

Evaluation is a very familiar term to nurse educators. Educators spend a great deal of time and effort in evaluation, from assessing student performance to that of curriculum appropriateness. One area requiring evaluation that is often neglected is teaching effectiveness. To help educators improve student learning activities, students should be afforded the opportunity to evaluate the teaching experience. This includes a review of curriculum, courses, and teaching methods, as well as an evaluation of the teaching effectiveness of the educator.

Student evaluations of teaching effectiveness can be accomplished through a formal mechanism such as a course evaluation or by informal comments and suggestions. Regardless of the vehicle used for evaluating faculty, the existence of such a procedure is vital to sound educational principles. Evaluation is discussed further in Chapter 11.

Exhibit 2–7 Teaching Plan

CLASS _____ SUBJECT _____ INSTRUCTOR _____ DATE _____

Lesson Purpose:	Critical elements to be included:	Methods: ___ demonstration ___ discussion ___ lecture ___ participation ___ questions/answers ___ role playing ___ dramatizations ___ simulations ___ other
Student Behavioral Objectives As a result of this lesson, the student will: *Action Verb* *Expected Learning*	Review items:	
	Related terminology:	Aids: ___ blackboard/bulletin board ___ films/filmstrips ___ video cassettes ___ slides ___ tapes/records ___ handouts ___ pamphlets ___ illustrations ___ models/anatomic charts
Content:	Useful analogies/examples:	

SUMMARY

Nurse educators must have a conceptual framework for teaching that includes learning and nursing theory. This foundation provides the basis for quality education applicable to professional nursing. Educators can no longer "teach the way they were taught," but must develop strong principles upon which to establish their methods and strategies of teaching. If educators have a general knowledge of past and present learning theories, they will have a sound basis for classroom and clinical instruction. Likewise, nurse educators should have a background of information about nursing theories in order to project the concept of nursing and professionalism.

It is the responsibility of the nurse educator to provide an educationally stimulating environment in which students can learn. In establishing this positive learning experience, nurse educators should consider the attitudes, beliefs, and values of the students and accept each student as a unique individual with worth and dignity and special needs. It is through this educational philosophy that students will achieve self-actualization and personal and professional growth.

NOTES

1. B.F. Skinner, *The Behavior of Organisms: An Experimental Analysis* (New York: Appleton-Century-Crofts, Inc., 1966).

2. Heinz Werner, *Comparative Psychology of Mental Development* (New York: International University Press, 1957).

3. Jean Piaget, *The Psychology of The Child* (New York: Basic Books, 1969).

4. Sigmund Freud, *A General Introduction to Psychoanalysis* (New York: Liveright, 1935).

5. Imogene Kind, *Toward a Theory For Nursing* (New York: John Wiley and Sons, 1971).

6. Martha E. Rogers, *An Introduction to The Theoretical Basis of Nursing* (Philadelphia: F.A. Davis, 1970).

7. Dorothy Johnson, "Development of Theory: A Requisite for Nursing as a Primary Health Profession," *Nursing Research* 23 (1974): 372–377.

8. Callista Roy, *Introduction to Nursing: An Adaptation Model* (Englewood Cliffs, N.J.: Prentice-Hall, 1982).

9. Ida Jean Orlando, *The Dynamic Nurse-Patient Relationship: Function, Process, and Principles* (New York: Putnam, 1961).

10. Myra E. Levine, *Introduction to Clinical Nursing* (Philadelphia: F.A. Davis, 1973).

11. Dorothea E. Orem, *Nursing: Concepts of Practice* (New York: McGraw-Hill, 1980), 13.

12. Loretta E. Heidgerken, *Teaching and Learning in Schools of Nursing* (Philadelphia: J.P. Lippincott, 1965), 166.

13. Benjamin S. Bloom et al., *Taxonomy of Educational Objectives: Handbook I: Cognitive Domain* (New York: David McKay, 1965).

14. R.H. Dave, "Psychomotor Levels," in *Developing and Writing Behavioral Objectives* (Tucson, Ariz.: Educational Innovators Press, 1970), 33.

15. Bruce W. Tuckman, "A Four-Domain Taxonomy for Classifying Educational Tasks and Objectives," *Educational Technology* 12 (December 1972): 36–38.

16. Elizabeth J. Simpson, "A Classification of Educational Objectives: Psychomotor Domain," *Illinois Teachers of Home Economics* 10 (1966): 110.

17. Helen S. O'Shea and Margaret K. Parsons, "Clinical Instruction: Effective and Ineffective Teacher Behaviors," *Nursing Outlook* 27 (June 1979): 411–415.

18. Carl R. Rogers, *Freedom To Learn* (Columbus, Oh.: Bell & Howell Co., 1969).

19. Phyllis J. Karns and Therese A. Schwab, "Therapeutic Communication and Clinical Instruction," *Nursing Outlook* 30 (January 1982): 39–43.

SUGGESTED READINGS

Bernard, Harold W. *Psychology of Learning and Teaching.* New York: McGraw-Hill, 1972.

Chinn, Peggy L. *Advances in Nursing Theory Development.* Rockville, Md.: Aspen Systems, 1983.

Conley, Virginia C. *Curriculum and Instruction in Nursing.* Boston: Little, Brown, 1973.

Dave. R.H. "Psychomotor Levels," in *Developing and Writing Behavioral Objectives.* Tucson, Ariz.: Educational Innovators Press, 1970.

deTornyay, Rheba. *Strategies For Teaching Nursing.* New York: John Wiley, 1971.

Evans, Richard I. *B.F. Skinner: The Man and His Ideas.* New York: Appleton-Century-Crofts, 1981.

————. *Carl Rogers: The Man and His Ideas.* New York: E.P. Dutton, 1975.

Guinee, Kathleen K. *Teaching and Learning in Nursing.* New York: Macmillan, 1978.

Heidgerken, Loretta E. *Teaching and Learning in Schools of Nursing.* Philadelphia: J.B. Lippincott, 1965.

Hilgard, Ernest R., and Gordon H. Bower. *Theories of Learning.* Englewood Cliffs, N.J.: Prentice-Hall, 1975.

Johnson, Dorothy E. "A Philosophy of Nursing." *Nursing Outlook* 7 (1959): 198–200.

————. "Development of Theory: A Requisite For Nursing as a Primary Health Profession." *Nursing Research* 23 (1974): 372–377.

Jones, J. Charles. *Learning.* New York: Harcourt, Brace & World, 1967.

Karns, Phyllis J., and Therese A. Schwab. "Therapeutic Communication and Clinical Instruction." *Nursing Outlook* 30 (January 1982): 39–43.

King, Imogene M. *Toward a Theory For Nursing.* New York: John Wiley, 1971.

Knowles, Malcolm S. *The Adult Education Movement in the United States.* New York: Holt, Rinehart & Winston, 1962.

Langer, Jonas. *Theories of Development.* New York: Holt, Rinehart & Winston, 1969.

Levine, Myra E. *Introduction to Clinical Nursing,* 2nd ed. Philadelphia: F.A. Davis, 1973.

Muse, Maude B. *Guiding Learning Experience.* New York: Macmillan, 1950.

Newman, Margaret. *Theory Development in Nursing.* Philadelphia: F.A. Davis, 1981.

Orem, Dorothea E. *Nursing: Concepts of Practice.* New York: McGraw-Hill, 1980.

Reilly, Dorothy E. *Behavioral Objectives—Evaluation in Nursing.* New York: Appleton-Century-Crofts, 1980.

Riehl, Joan P., and Callista Roy. *Conceptual Model for Nursing Practice.* New York: Appleton-Century-Crofts, 1980.

Rogers, Martha E. *An Introduction to the Theoretical Basis of Nursing*. Philadelphia: F.A. Davis, 1970.

Simpson, Elizabeth J. *A Classification of Educational Objectives: Psychomotor Domain*. Mt. Rainier, Md.: Gryphon Press, 1972.

Stevens, Barbara J. *Nursing Theory*. Boston: Little, Brown, 1979.

The Nursing Theories Conference Group. *Nursing Theories: The Base for Professional Nursing Practice*. Englewood Cliffs, N.J.: Prentice-Hall, 1980.

Tuckman, Bruce W. "A Four-Domain Taxonomy for Classifying Educational Tasks and Objectives." *Educational Technology* 12 (December 1972): 36–38.

Wadsworth, Barry J. *Piaget's Theory of Cognitive Development*. New York: David McKay, 1972.

Werner, Heinz. "The Concept of Development From a Comparative and Organismic Point of View." In *Readings in Child Behavior and Development,* edited by C.S. Lavatelli and F. Stendler. New York: Harcourt Brace Jovanovich, 1972, 47–54.

Wlodkowski, Raymond J. *Motivation*. Washington D.C.: National Education Association, 1977.

Appendix 2–A

Behavioral Verbs Appropriate for Each Level of the Three Taxonomies

I. Cognitive
  C1.0 Information

define	name
identify	recall
list	recognize

  C2.0 Comprehension
      C2.1 Translation level

cite examples of	give in own words

      C2.2 Interpretation level

choose	discriminate
demonstrate use of	explain
describe	interpret
differentiate	select

      C2.3 Extrapolation level

conclude	estimate
detect	infer
determine	predict
draw conclusions	

  C3.0 Application

apply	generalize
develop	relate
employ	use

  C4.0 Analysis

appraise	detect
compare	distinguish

Source: Dorothy E. Reilly, *Behavioral Objectives—Evaluation in Nursing*. New York: Appleton-Century-Crofts, Inc., © 1980. Reprinted with permission.

contrast   evaluate
criticize   identify
deduce
C5.0 Synthesis
classify   produce
design   reconstruct
develop   restructure
modify   synthesize
organize   systematize
C6.0 Evaluation
appraise   evaluate
assess   judge
critique   validate

II. Affective
A1.0 Receiving
acknowledges   shows awareness of
shares
A2.0 Responding
acts willingly   practices
discusses willingly   responds
expresses satisfaction in   seeks opportunities
is willing to support   selects
listens to   shows interest
A3.0 Valuing
accepts   cooperates with
acclaims   helps
agrees   participates in
assists   respects
assumes responsibility   supports
A4.0 Organization of Values
argues   formulates a position
debates   is consistent
declares   takes a stand
defends
A5.0 Characterization by Value
acts consistently   stands for
is accountable

III. Psychomotor Behaviors According to Taxonomy
P1.0 Imitation
follows example of
follows lead of

P2.0 Manipulation
         carries out according   follows procedure
         to procedure   practices
P3.0 Precision
         demonstrates skill in using
P4.0 Articulation
         carries out   uses
         is skillful in using
P5.0 Naturalization
         is competent   carries out
         is skilled

Chapter 3

Accountability and Clinical Instruction

Accountability in the health professions became a very popular and controversial issue in the 1970s. As consumers have demanded better health care, the burden of responsibility for its provision has fallen equally on all members of the health team. As the major professions in health care, both medicine and nursing must assume maximum responsibility for the quality of care available to the public. Within this framework, the issue of accountability takes on greater meaning for both professions.

Accountability is defined in Webster's unabridged dictionary as "the quality or state of being accountable, liable and responsible."[1] Another definition from Webster states that to be accountable means "to be answerable." These definitions suggest that someone other than oneself judges the degree of fulfillment of specified obligations. Thus, individuals are held accountable by someone for all their actions. To whom one is accountable depends on what one is accountable for. When discussing the phenomenon of accountability, one must ask: Accountable for what? And to whom?

Broadly speaking, accountability in the nursing profession means providing a nursing service according to set priorities. In order for an individual to be held accountable or responsible for a nursing action, a safety or quality standard must exist as a criterion of measurement. The nurse can be held liable for only those nursing activities for which performance competencies have been developed.

ACCOUNTABILITY AND THE CONSUMER

In 1975 the Congress for Nursing Practice of the American Nurses' Association recognized its responsibility to the health consumer to improve nursing practice by formulating its Standards for Nursing Practice. These standards are based on the nursing process and provide a baseline for determining quality nursing care. This

31

accomplishment of the American Nurses' Association fulfilled the obligation of the nursing profession to monitor nursing care. The generic standards are a broadly stated document that focuses on general nursing practice. It consists of the eight standards listed in Exhibit 3–1, each with appropriate rationale followed by assessment factors.

The Standards for Nursing Practice can be applied to nursing practice in any clinical setting. Separate standards exist for the following areas: community health, maternal and child health, mental health, orthopedic nursing, operating room, emergency room, cardiovascular nursing, geriatric nursing, nursing service, continued education, and nursing education. Because even the specific standards provide only a baseline from which to act, the professional nurse must assume responsibility for individualization and implementation of nursing care.

Accountability entails both legal and ethical obligations of nursing. It is inherent to professionalism and must be viewed as both a legal and an ethical duty. Monitoring professional practice should come from within the profession by the appropriate groups or individuals. Thus, the second aspect of accountability deals with the question: Accountable to whom?

Legally, the nursing profession is accountable to state registration laws called nurse practice acts. Nurse practice acts did not exist prior to the 1900s, when any training nurses received was informal and their role was simply that of a physician's assistant. It was not until the early 1900s that several states passed nursing laws establishing rules and regulations for nursing education and licensure that

---

Exhibit 3–1 ANA Standards for Nursing Practice

Standard 1	The collection of data about the health status of the client/patient is systematic and continuous. The data are accessible, communicated, and recorded.
Standard 2	*Nursing diagnoses* are derived from health status data.
Standard 3	The *plan of nursing care* includes *goals* derived from nursing diagnoses.
Standard 4	The plan of nursing care includes *priorities* and the prescribed nursing approaches or measures to achieve the goals derived from the nursing diagnoses.
Standard 5	*Nursing actions* provide for client/patient participation in health promotion, maintenance, and restoration.
Standard 6	Nursing actions assist the client/patient to maximize his health capabilities.
Standard 7	The client/patient's progress or lack of progress toward goal achievement is determined by the client/patient and the nurse.
Standard 8	The client/patient's progress or lack of progress toward goal achievement directs reassessment, reordering of priorities, new goal setting, and revision of the plan of nursing care.

Source: Congress for Nursing Practice of the American Nurses' Association. *Standards for Nursing Practice* (Kansas City, Mo.: ANA, 1975). Reprinted with permission.

governed methods for administering the law and creating state boards of nursing. In March 1903 the first registration act (nurse practice act) was passed in North Carolina.[2] This began a progressive movement in nursing as each state campaigned to pass similar laws. By 1923 all states in the union as well as Washington, D.C., and Hawaii had nurse practice acts.[3] These original state acts did not include a definition of nursing since the nurse still functioned within the realm of medicine. In 1938 New York included the following definition in its Nurse Practice Act:

A person practices nursing within the meaning of this article who for compensation or personal profit (a) performs any professional service requiring the applications of principles of nursing based on biological, physical and social sciences, such as responsible supervision of a patient requiring skill in observation of symptoms and reactions and the accurate recording of the facts and carrying out of treatments and medications as prescribed by a licensed physician, and the application of such nursing procedures as involve understanding of cause and others; or (b) performs such duties as are required in the physical care of a patient and in carrying out of medical orders as prescribed by a licensed physician, requiring an understanding of nursing but not requiring the professional service as outlined in (a).[4]

In 1955 the American Nurses' Association adopted the following model definition of nursing:

The practice of professional nursing means the performance for compensation of any act in the observation, care and counsel of the ill, injured, or infirm, or in the maintenance of health or prevention of illness of others, or in the supervision and teaching of other personnel, or the administration of medications and treatments prescribed by a licensed physician or dentist; requiring substantial specialized judgment and skill and based on knowledge and application of the principles of biological, physical and social sciences. The foregoing shall not be deemed to include acts of diagnosis or prescription of therapeutic or corrective measures.[5]

These definitions demonstrate the limited scope of the practice of nursing from the onset of formal legislation until the middle fifties. The changes that have occurred in nursing since the fifties were the direct result of the women's rights movement and the national shortage of nurses. The following statement, added to the American Nurses' Association definition in 1970, typifies the changes that have occurred in the field of nursing:

A professional nurse may also perform such additional acts, under emergency or other special conditions, which may include special training, as are recognized by the medical and nursing professions as proper to be performed by a professional nurse under such conditions, even though such acts might otherwise be considered diagnosis and prescription.[6]

As the role of nursing expanded to meet the increased needs of the health consumer, states had to change their nurse practice acts to keep pace. The state of Washington revised its nurse practice act to define nursing as

the performance of acts requiring substantial specialized knowledge, judgment and skill based upon the principles of the biological, physiological, behavioral and sociological sciences in either:

(1) The observation, assessment, diagnosis, care or counsel, and health teaching of the ill, injured, or infirm, or in the maintenance of health or prevention of illness in others.

(2) The performance of such additional acts requiring education and training and which are recognized jointly by the medical and nursing professions as proper to be performed by nurses licensed under this chapter and which shall be authorized by the board of nursing through its rules and regulations.

(3) The administration, supervision, delegation, and evaluation of nursing practice; PROVIDED, HOWEVER, that nothing herein shall affect the authority of any hospital, hospital district, medical clinic or office, concerning its administration and supervision.

(4) The teaching of nursing.

(5) The executing of medical regimen as prescribed by a licensed physician, dentist, or chiropodist.[7]

Comparing the definition of nursing quoted earlier from the 1938 New York nurse practice act with the following present-day definition shows the vast differences between nursing in the past and nursing in the present:

The practice of the profession of nursing as a registered professional nurse is defined as diagnosing and treating human responses to actual or potential health problems through such services as case finding, health teaching, health counseling, and provision of care supportive to or restorative of life and well-being, and executing medical regimens as prescribed by a licensed or otherwise legally authorized physician or dentist. A nursing regimen shall be consistent with and shall not vary any existing medical regimen.[8]

These two nurse practice acts demonstrate the degree to which nursing has changed since the nursing profession has been held legally accountable for good-quality nursing practice. Nurse practice acts provide the foundation for nursing within each state as they define nursing practice and supply a basis for legal accountability. Most nurse practice acts include (1) a definition of nursing, (2) creation of the state board of nurse examiners, (3) responsibilities and composition of the board, (4) licensure requirements, (5) licensure exemption, (6) licensure revocation, (7) licensure reciprocity with other states, and (8) penalties for practicing without a license. The primary purpose of these nursing laws is to protect the health care consumer from incompetent nursing practitioners. They regulate nursing practice and hold professional nurses accountable to practice nursing according to the definition within the law.

To whom are nurses ethically accountable? Many nurse practice acts state explicitly that the nurse is accountable to the health consumer. According to the Washington State nurse practice act, "The registered nurse is directly accountable and responsible to the individual consumer for the quality of nursing care rendered."[9] Although this nurse practice act projects the trends of nursing and its role in providing health care, accountability is not a new concept to the nursing profession.

As early as 1950 nursing recognized its responsibility to the health care consumer when the American Nurses' Association adopted the Code of Ethics for Nurses (see Exhibit 3–2). Ethics are value judgments that label conduct as right or wrong. Ethical behavior is a moral obligation as opposed to a legal one imposed by law. The Code of Ethics for Nurses serves as a guide for behaving professionally and meeting the standards of nursing practice with personal moral accountability for one's own actions.

Although there is no legal basis for the code's statements, the nursing profession relies upon the standards for identifying unethical behavior and determining the consequences of such conduct. Nursing licenses have been revoked by the profession when individuals have behaved in direct contradiction to the Code of Ethics for Nurses. Through this code, the nursing profession accepts the responsibility for policing the behavior of its members in regard to their ethical conduct.

Since 1950 the American Nurses' Association has periodically updated its code of ethics. The code defines basic human rights and the responsibility of the professional nurse to uphold these rights as shown in Exhibit 3–2.

The ANA's Code of Ethics not only identifies the responsibility of nursing to provide competent nursing services, but also describes specific nursing care that

Exhibit 3–2 ANA Code of Ethics for Nurses

1. The nurse provides services with respect for human dignity and the uniqueness of the client unrestricted by considerations of social or economic status, personal attributes, or the nature of health problems.
2. The nurse safeguards the client's right to privacy by judiciously protecting information of a confidential nature.
3. The nurse acts to safeguard the client and the public when health care and safety are affected by the incompetent, unethical, or illegal practice of any person.
4. The nurse assumes responsibility and accountability for individual nursing judgments and actions.
5. The nurse maintains competence in nursing.
6. The nurse exercises informed judgment and uses individual competence and qualifications as criteria in seeking consultation, accepting responsibilities, and delegating nursing activities to others.
7. The nurse participates in activities that contribute to the ongoing development of the profession's body of knowledge.
8. The nurse participates in the profession's efforts to implement and improve standards of nursing.
9. The nurse participates in the profession's efforts to establish and maintain conditions of employment conducive to high quality nursing care.
10. The nurse participates in the profession's effort to protect the public from misinformation and misrepresentation and to maintain the integrity of nursing.
11. The nurse collaborates with members of the health professions and other citizens in promoting community and national efforts to meet the health needs of the public.

Source: American Nurses' Association. *The Code for Nurses.* rev. ed. (Kansas City, Mo.: ANA, 1976). Reprinted with permission.

each client has a right to expect. This mention of clients' rights occurred long before the publication of the Patient's Bill of Rights by the American Hospital Association (AHA) in 1972 (see Exhibit 3–3). Whether a physician chooses to endorse the client rights and incorporate them in medical practice is a personal decision. However, common law (law based on court rules) has established that the physician is legally accountable to the health consumer for actions included in the Patient's Bill of Rights.

The Pennsylvania Nurses' Association (PNA) Commission on Nursing Practice developed a document supporting the client's right to quality care, *Consumer's Rights to Nursing Care*, published in 1979 (see Exhibit 3–4). Besides supporting the 12 rights identified by the American Hospital Association, this document affirms the importance of the client's own values and affirms the role of the nurse as an advocate for the client. The latter demonstrates the willingness of the nursing profession to accept the responsibility for protecting clients' rights.

Exhibit 3–3 AHA Patient's Bill of Rights

1. The patient has the right to considerate and respectful care.
2. The patient has the right to obtain from his physician complete current information concerning his diagnosis, treatment, and prognosis in terms the patient can be reasonably expected to understand. When it is not medically advisable to give such information to the patient, the information should be made available to an appropriate person in his behalf. He has the right to know by the name the physician responsible for coordinating his care.
3. The patient has the right to receive from his physician information necessary to give informed consent prior to the start of any procedure and/or treatment. Except in emergencies, such information for informed consent should include but not necessarily be limited to the specific procedure and/or treatment, the medically significant risks involved, and the probable duration of incapacitation. Where medically significant alternatives for care or treatment exist, or when the patient requests information concerning medical alternatives, the patient has the right to such information. The patient also has the right to know the name of the person responsible for the procedures and/or treatment.
4. The patient has the right to refuse treatment to the extent permitted by law, and to be informed of the medical consequences of his action.
5. The patient has the right to every consideration of his privacy concerning his own medical care program. Case discussion, consultation, examination, and treatment are confidential and should be conducted discreetly. Those not directly involved in his care must have the permission of the patient to be present.
6. The patient has the right to expect that all communications and records pertaining to his care should be treated as confidential.
7. The patient has the right to expect that within its capacity a hospital must make reasonable response to the request of a patient for services. The hospital must provide evaluation, service, and/or referral as indicated by the urgency of the case. When medically permissible a patient may be transferred to another facility only after he has received complete information and explanation concerning the needs for and alternatives to such a transfer. The institution to which the patient is to be transferred must first have accepted the patient for transfer.
8. The patient has the right to obtain information as to any relationship of his hospital to other health care and educational institutions insofar as his care is concerned. The patient has the right to obtain information as to the existence of any professional relationships among individuals, by name, who are treating him.
9. The patient has the right to be advised if the hospital proposes to engage in or perform human experimentation affecting his care or treatment. The patient has the right to refuse to participate in such research projects.
10. The patient has the right to expect reasonable continuity of care. He has the right to know in advance what appointment times and physicians are available and where. The patient has the right to expect that the hospital will provide a mechanism whereby he is informed by his physician or a delegate of the physician of the patient's continuing health.
11. The patient has the right to examine and receive an explanation of his bill regardless of source of payment.
12. The patient has the right to know what hospital rules and regulations apply to his conduct as a patient.

Source: American Hospital Association. *A Patient's Bill of Rights* (Chicago: AHA, 1972). Reprinted with the permission of the American Hospital Association. Copyright 1972.

Exhibit 3–4 PNA Consumer's Rights to Nursing Care

You [the client] have the right to:

1. Receive nursing care regardless of race, religion, sex, national origin, age, life style, ability to pay or source of payment.
2. Be treated with dignity, respect, and courtesy.
3. Be greeted by name and to receive an explanation of agency routine, policies and facilities where appropriate.
4. Proper identification of the registered nurse and other nursing personnel by name and title.
5. Care provided by nursing personnel who are qualified, through education, experience and training, to carry out the services for which they are responsible.
6. Be informed of the tentative plan for your nursing care, including an explanation of procedures and medication.
7. Have an opportunity to discuss with a registered nurse your needs (physical, emotional, and spiritual) and to participate, along with your family, in your individualized nursing care.
8. Continuity of all necessary services throughout the period of your need. This could include the use of appropriate personnel within and outside the health care agency and community resources.
9. Privacy and confidentiality in all aspects of your nursing care.
10. Receive needed health care teaching and/or counselling that you can understand.
11. Receive medications and treatments as ordered by your physician with appropriate explanations.
12. Expect the registered nurse to respond to your right to refuse any aspect of your health care.
13. Expect the registered nurse to respond to your questions regarding any aspect of your care.
14. Expect the registered nurse to be responsible for informing your physician of changes in your condition.
15. Basic nursing care including concern for personal hygiene and safety, nutrition, activity, rest, and comfort according to your needs.
16. Respect for your values, including those involving life or death.
17. Expect the registered nurse to be your advocate.

Source: Pennsylvania Nurses' Association. Commission on Nursing Practice. *Consumer Rights to Nursing Care* (Harrisburg, Pa.: PNA, 1979). Reprinted with permission.

ETHICAL RESPONSIBILITY

Whereas the professional nurse is held accountable to the law for providing safe nursing care to the consumer, ethical accountability is a personal responsibility that nurses and all other health professionals must accept. Protecting the rights of the client who has entered the health care system is a responsibility the professional nurse shares with others in the medical professions. As the client's advocate, the professional nurse is obligated to coordinate the health services provided to the client by all members of the health team. Every professional nurse has a responsibility to the health care consumer to base his or her nursing practice upon the ethical standards identified by the profession. As legal and ethical accountability are established by the consumer in the courtroom, the nursing profession is challenged to meet the demand for high-quality care with nursing excellence.

NURSING EDUCATION

Accountability is not new in education, but its requirements since the 1970s provided nurse educators with many challenges. Societal trends have dictated that nursing educators be accountable for preparing competent and safe practitioners of nursing. They are also held responsible for providing safe nursing care to consumers during the process. The client, once viewed as a passive recipient of health care, is now seen as an active consumer of health care services. Students also have become active participants in the social system, demanding their rights as consumers of education. Institutions of higher learning and nursing educators are now being held accountable for providing good-quality education and quality nursing care. In nursing education, accountability must be shared three ways, directly involving the institution, the educator, and the nursing student or graduate.

The Educational Institution

Although the primary responsibility of the nursing school is to its students and faculty, it is also accountable to state and federal governments. All types of governmental rules regulate institutions and service-oriented programs. The educational facility must be held accountable to specific departments within governmental agencies on both the state and the federal level. Whether they provide funding for the educational institution or are regulatory bodies supervising the institution's educational mission, these agencies hold institutions of higher learning accountable to them for their varied functions.

One of the major benefits of the consumer advocacy movement in the nation has been the improvement of all educational programs. The consumer has become involved in all aspects of social and educational reform—in the process as well as product of the educational system. One method of assessing the quality of education provided by an institution is for the institution to complete a self-evaluation study and determine where changes for improvement should be made. Another is to seek national accreditation voluntarily from appropriate accrediting agencies. National accreditation reaps monetary benefits for the institution as well as serving as proof that it can provide sound and effective education for potential students. Many grants, loans, and scholarships are based on the accreditation status of the institution. Since the educational criteria designated by the national agency must be met before achieving accreditation, high-quality education is ensured. Seeking accreditation assures students that the institution is accepting responsibility for providing the best possible educational opportunities.

Once an educational institution assumes the responsibility for a nursing program it must support it to maintain accountability to the student. The institution has contractual obligations to provide the course offerings and counseling and academic, health, and tutorial services it lists in its catalog. These are contractual because they are stated in the college catalog. The institution that offers a professional nursing program has made a commitment to provide students with the facilities and equipment needed to meet the curriculum objectives. As consumers of the institution's educational services, students must be provided with teachers and learning opportunities they need to fulfill the objectives of the program.

The institution's responsibility to the educator is to ensure academic freedom, fulfill mutual expectations, and provide program support. Nursing faculty should function within the institution under the same rules and regulations as other faculty. The instructor should be given freedom in the classroom and clinical setting to discuss the educational material in the manner in which he or she chooses. Within this freedom, however, the educator has the responsibility for selecting and organizing the learning experiences that are appropriate for meeting the specific course objectives.

The mutual expectations of the institution and the faculty should be discussed and reviewed by both parties. Airing of ideas and expectations provides a sound basis for evaluation. Many colleges and universities require that a contract be written between faculty member and institution at the time of employment stating mutual expectations as illustrated in Exhibit 3–5.

The institution must be accountable for support of the nursing program in providing a working budget, appropriate equipment, adequate facilities, sufficient personnel, and so on. Educating professional nurses is an expensive proposition and does not always produce tangible financial results. The numerous institutional problems that often result may filter down to the students, affecting their learning experience. The institution must be accountable to provide high-quality education regardless of political and financial concerns if it has made the commitment to do so.

The Nurse Educator

The nurse educator's responsibility to the institution is to offer high-quality instruction through a sound and well-defined curriculum. The instructor's accountability involves a commitment to provide nursing education within the framework of the educational system that meets the goals and objectives of the institution. Nursing education is responsible to the institution of higher learning for partial fulfillment of its mission. Thus, it is imperative that the philosophy and

Exhibit 3–5 Faculty Employment Contract

I. As an employee of this institution, I plan to
  A. Provide educational experiences to assist students in meeting program objectives.
  B. Be available with specific office hours and/or other individual arrangements for
    1. Academic guidance.
    2. Personal counseling.
  C. Participate in
    1. College committees inter- and intradepartmentally.
    2. Campus activities.
    3. Community affairs representing the college and department in advisory and educational capacities.
  D. Be available to present continuing education programs special to my expertise.
  E. Continue my education toward a masters in nursing and a doctorate in nursing so that I am better equipped
    1. In the philosophies of my dual professions—nursing and education—and to develop further knowledge in these professions.
    2. To assist and teach nursing students at _____.
    3. To discuss, research, prepare, and possibly publish materials regarding concepts within the fields of nursing and health education.
  F. Attend workshops, special programs, and conventions in order to increase my abilities and give assistance to students.
  G. Maintain membership in professional organizations in order to
    1. Keep abreast of new concepts and materials.
    2. Represent the college and foster better understanding between the college and organizations.
    3. Support the organizations to obtain better working conditions.
    4. Represent the organization in fostering better understanding between the public and profession.
II. As an employee of this institution, I expect the college to provide
  A. Academic freedom.
  B. Adequate supervision and appropriate leadership from my peers and administration.
  C. Reasonable working environment and conditions, such as
    1. Individual office space in order to
      a. Interview, counsel, and advise students in privacy.
      b. Provide maximum output of materials for the college.
    2. Aesthetic environment in order to function to maximum capacity, e.g., window, heat, dry area, periodic painting of walls.
  D. Adequate office supplies and supportive and audio-visual aids to provide maximum output.
  E. Reimbursement for courses taken to further my education.
  F. Monetary assistance for meaningful workshops and programs as determined by the nursing department, which would further my ability to assist, advise, and teach students.
  G. Time, with monetary assistance, to complete residential requirements toward a doctorate degree.

objectives of the nursing curriculum be consistent with the core curriculum and the philosophy and objectives of the institution.

The nursing faculty must be actively involved in designing, developing, and implementing a curriculum that is well constructed and workable. The nurse educator must view this task as important to the instructor and the student, as well as to nursing. Curriculum development is an important aspect of accountability because it directly affects the institution, the educator, the student, and the client. The philosophy and objectives must be derived from the philosophy and objectives of the institution, so that the institution demonstrates consistency between its goals and the goals of the educational programs.

The student must also support the curriculum and its framework in order for the learning process to be effective. If the philosophy views students as active participants in their own education, students must reciprocate by taking the initiative in learning and including self-direction, independent study, and self-evaluation in their life experiences.

The educator too must be an active participant of the philosophy and must support the philosophy, objectives, and conceptual framework of the nursing program in order to provide the student with quality education. The nurse educator who does not believe in the philosophy and conceptual framework specified by the nursing program that employs him or her but will comply with it should evaluate his or her own effectiveness as a teacher in that nursing program. In order for an educator to support a specific curriculum during the teaching process, he or she must internalize the concepts and principles held valuable by the nursing faculty. Without this prizing of the program's philosophy and conceptual framework, the educator will not function in the best possible manner, and teaching competencies will be lower. The nurse educator also has responsibility to the institution to demonstrate knowledge of the subject matter as well as expertise in the art of clinical instruction. In addition to classroom instruction and clinical supervision, the nurse educator usually has other areas of responsibility. Duties usually identifed in the faculty job description include academic advisement, departmental and institutional committee membership and activities, personal counseling, continued education, publication, and research. Exhibit 3–6 is a sample job description for a position as associate professor.

Accountability for job functions such as those described in Exhibit 3–6 is usually measured by a peer evaluation system based on specified criteria. Typical evaluation criteria would be the following:

1. Appropriate instructional methods
2. Integration of appropriate teaching aids
3. Expertise in subject matter
4. Enthusiasm for subject matter
5. Sharing of knowledge in areas of expertise

Exhibit 3–6 Job Description for a Nursing Faculty Position

---

1. Instructs, supervises, and evaluates students in the nursing courses under the direction of the chairman of the nursing department.
2. Plans, reviews, and revises the nursing curriculum.
3. Develops and maintains current course outlines for courses for which he or she is responsible.
4. Meets with nursing personnel of cooperating agencies to interpret course and program objectives to plan for clinical experiences.
5. Serves as a resource person, upon request, to the nursing staff of the cooperating agencies.
6. Acts as a resource person to other faculty members in area of clinical specialization or theoretical competency.
7. Communicates regularly with non-nurse faculty members to promote understanding and continuity of the program.
8. Communicates regularly with nursing instructors and offers assistance when needed.
9. Serves as counselor to students having personal or academic problems and refers them to the college guidance center or the mental health center when indicated.
10. Acts as an adviser to students as they plan their courses to meet degree requirements.
11. Participates in student-parent/spouse conferences.
12. Interviews and gives guidance to possible candidates for the nursing program.
13. Assists in screening applicants for nurse faculty positions.
14. Orients new faculty to course and course materials.
15. Attends general and departmental faculty meetings.
16. Accepts speaking engagements in relation to nursing.
17. Performs as an active member of nursing and related organizations.
18. Attends professional meetings and participates in their activities.

---

6. Availability for student advisement
7. Rapport with co-workers
8. Continued professional growth and involvement in

- Research
- Scholarship
- Professional contributions
- Professional organizations
- Local health programs

9. Participation in college faculty programs
10. Participation in nursing faculty organization
11. Professional involvement in departmental committees and programs
12. Student evaluation

Each of the criteria listed would need to be addressed with specific behavioral objectives in order to measure their achievement.

Other more technical areas of accountability include office hours, work hours, teaching load, student/teacher ratios, contact hours, and so on. It is important that each nurse educator be made aware of his or her responsibility to the institution and the department before being held accountable. The procedure for informing new faculty of responsibilities and expectations can be incorporated into orientation.

The nurse educator has professional responsibility to the institution to develop academic procedures and policies. Since the procedures and policies may affect the students during the education process, the nursing instructor also has a personal responsibility to students to inform them of these procedures and policies in easily understandable terms. Students should understand the grading system and the consequences of failure. Having information such as the processes for dismissal and readmission in a written policy protects the institution from litigation as well as providing students with a clear picture of their role in the educational process. Other policies that should be made explicit are those on the evaluation process, leaves of absence, maternity leave, and student employment.

Total curriculum evaluation is one method of ensuring that good-quality education is being provided by the nursing faculty. This self-evaluation should be an automatic process that helps the nurse educators identify the strengths and weaknesses of the nursing program. It is only by recognizing deficiencies of the curriculum and making appropriate adjustments that the quality of nursing education can be improved. Exhibit 3–7 is a sample of a curriculum evaluation plan.

Student Rights

The nurse educator should be aware of the laws and programs that provide for or protect the rights of the student in the nursing program. As a consumer of nursing education, the student has specific rights that must be valued as important by the nurse educator. The nurse educator must be knowledgeable about these student rights and the issues relating to student accountability in order to understand how to comply.

Accountability and the rights of students first became an important issue in the 1960s. Since that time laws and programs have been legislated in an effort to provide quality education for students while maintaining their basic rights. In March 1974 the Education Commission of the United States held the first conference on student rights and quality education. As a result of a follow-up conference in November of the same year, suggestions were made concerning rights and responsibilities of the student in institutions of higher learning.

In April 1975 the National Student Nurses' Association (NSNA) adopted the Student Bill of Rights, which includes 20 statements relating to the rights of nursing students (see Exhibit 3–8). These rights touch all aspects of student life, both academic and personal. They are important for the nursing student as well as

Exhibit 3–7 Curriculum Evaluation Plan

A systematic plan of evaluation has been developed by which each aspect of the department and the educational program will be evaluated. Following each semester, a day will be designated for this curriculum evaluation.

I. The following aspects will be evaluated at the end of each Fall semester:
  A. Nonacademic programs
    1. Health
    2. Counseling
    3. Advisement
  B. Facilities
    1. College
    2. Clinical
  C. Handbook
    1. Faculty
    2. Student
  D. Policies
    1. Faculty
    2. Student
  E. Curriculum
    1. National League for Nursing (NLN) achievement test
    2. State board examination
    3. Follow-up
II. The following aspects will be evaluated at the end of each Spring semester:
  A. Committees
  B. Records and reports
  C. Facilities
    1. College
    2. Clinical
  D. Guidelines for evaluation program
    1. Students
      a. Anecdotals
      b. Evaluation form
      c. Grading system
    2. Faculty
      a. Peer evaluation
      b. Student evaluation
    3. Courses
      a. Faculty
      b. Students
    4. Educational materials
      a. Texts
      b. Audiovisuals
  E. Curriculum
    1. Review and revise
      a. Philosophy
      b. Curriculum objectives
      c. Conceptual framework themes

Exhibit 3–7 continued

> 2. Trace themes through the following:
>   a. Philosophy
>   b. Curriculum objectives
>   c. Level objectives
>   d. Course objectives
>   e. Unit objectives
>   f. Class objectives
>   g. Text
> 3. Review and revise courses
>   a. Relation to Curriculum
>   b. Content
>   c. Clinical Experience
>   d. Tests
> F. Students
>   1. Methods used to evaluate student progress through the program
>   a. Classroom evaluation through student participation in discussion, written tests, reports
>   b. Evaluation of clinical performance report by instructor(s)
>   c. Personal supervision and conferences with instructors
>   2. Opportunities of students for self-evaluation
>   a. Students write anecdotal notes and utilize these in writing their self-evaluation reports
>   b. Opportunity to write comments on evaluation report written by the instructor
>   3. Opportunities for students to assist in evaluating their respective educational programs
>   a. Opportunity to write evaluations of various aspects of their experiences to be utilized by faculty in planning future experiences
>   b. Written evaluations of courses and instructors

the nurse educator and should be incorporated into the policies and procedures of every nursing program.

The nursing instructor also has a responsibility to students to provide the instruction needed by them to meet the goals and objectives of the curriculum. As consumers of nursing education, the students have invested time, energy, and finances in an educational process that must offer them information and training vital to their future as professional nurses. They hope that the program will provide them with the knowledge needed to pass the state board's examinations as well as the competencies needed to provide good-quality care to clients. The nursing faculty as a whole is accountable for giving students the opportunity to accomplish these goals.

In recent years the larger number of health care consumers have been living and working in the community instead of hospitalized in acute care agencies. In re-

Exhibit 3–8 NSNA Student's Bill of Rights

1. Students should be encouraged to develop the capacity for critical judgment and engage in a sustained and independent search for truth.

2. The freedom to teach and the freedom to learn are inseparable facets of academic freedom: students should exercise their freedom with responsibility.

3. Each institution has a duty to develop policies and procedures which provide and safeguard the students' freedom to learn.

4. Under no circumstances should a student be barred from admission to a particular institution on the basis of race, creed, sex, or marital status.

5. Students should be free to take reasoned exception to the data or views offered in any course of study and to reserve judgment about matters of opinion, but they are responsible for learning the content of any course of study for which they are enrolled.

6. Students should have protection through orderly procedures against prejudiced or capricious academic evaluation, but they are responsible for maintaining standards of academic performance established for each course in which they are enrolled.

7. Information about student views, beliefs, and political associations which instructors acquire in the course of their work should be considered confidential and not released without the knowledge or consent of the student.

8. The student should have the right to have a responsible voice in the determination of his/her curriculum.

9. Institutions should have a carefully considered policy as to the information which should be a part of a student's permanent educational record and as to the conditions of this disclosure.

10. Students and student organizations should be free to examine and discuss all questions of interest to them, and to express opinions publicly and privately.

11. Students should be allowed to invite and to hear any person of their own choosing, thereby taking the responsibility of furthering their education.

12. The student body should have clearly defined means to participate in the formulation and application of institutional policy affecting academic and student affairs.

13. The institution has an obligation to clarify those standards of behavior which it considers essential to its educational mission and its community life.

14. Disciplinary proceedings should be instituted only for violations of standards of conduct formulated with significant student participation and published in advance through such means as a student handbook or a generally available body of institutional regulations. It is the responsibility of the student to know these regulations. Grievance procedures should be available for every student.

15. As citizens and members of an academic community, students are subject to the obligations which accrue them by virtue of this membership and should enjoy the same freedoms of citizenship.

16. Students have the right to belong or refuse to belong to any organization of their choice.

17. Students have the right to personal privacy in their living space to the extent that the welfare of others is respected.

18. Adequate safety precautions should be provided by schools of nursing, for example, to and from student dorms, adequate street lighting, locks, etc.

Exhibit 3–8 continued

19. Dress code, if present in school, should be established by student government in conjunction with the school director and faculty, so the highest professional standards possible are maintained, but also taking into consideration points of comfort and practicality for the student.
20. Grading systems should be carefully reviewed periodically with students and faculty for clarification and better student-faculty understanding.

Source: National Student Nurses' Association. *Student's Bill of Rights* (New York: NSNA, April 1975). Reprinted with permission.

sponse to societal trends, nursing education programs have begun to expand their clinical settings to include numerous community experiences. Many educational programs have moved most of their clinical effort into community settings. Although this move seems appropriate in theory, the fact remains that most nurses do work, after graduation, in acute care settings. Providing the nursing student with unrealistic amounts of community health experience while decreasing quality and quantity of clinical practice in acute care settings could have disastrous results. This approach to nursing education would fail to provide students with the knowledge and competencies that they would most likely need to be employable. Idealism without realism is a luxury that nursing educators cannot afford. Students who are educated without the skills and techniques and medical knowledge they may possibly need will find it impossible to function effectively in the "real" world.

Statements 1–3, 10, and 11 in the Student's Bill of Rights concern the responsibility of the nursing educator to safeguard the students' rights of freedom in the learning process. Mereness identified six freedoms related to student learning. They are the freedom to disagree, explore ideas, help choose educational goals, study independently, experiment, and know faculty.[10] The educator must provide students with learning experiences that will assist them in learning creatively by exploration and experimentation. Independent learning should be encouraged as a method of assisting students in making appropriate educational decisions and judgments. Finally, as a nurse educator one should give of oneself to benefit the nursing students, being available for student conferences and meetings to deal with student concerns and problems in an empathetic and caring manner.

The education and socialization of students in nursing can be augmented by faculty members who permit students to know them as people. Too often nurse educators present the practice of nursing as an exclusive means for self-actualization. Faculty, in their reluctance to share their personal lives with students, perpetuate this misconception. Informal "rap" sessions can provide students and faculty with the opportunity for dialogue that would otherwise not be possible in the structured curriculum.

The Student's Bill of Rights also includes items related to the personal freedom of the student. It supports the student's privacy in personal life, as a member of the community and a student of nursing. It directs the nursing program to establish safety precautions related to institutional facilities, equipment, and grounds. Joint accountability for dress codes is stressed, since both the nursing students and the nursing faculty should support the high standards of the nursing profession. Statements 15–19 convey to the educator his or her responsibility in supporting the personal freedom of the nursing student.

Statement 4 in the Student's Bill of Rights speaks to the issue of discrimination in the admission process of the institution. These issues have been legally supported by Title VI of the Civil Rights Act and Title IX of the Education Amendments. Racial discrimination has been illegal since 1954 when the U.S. Supreme Court supported integration and ruled that separate schools for children of different races were illegal. Title VI of the Civil Rights Act of 1964 prohibits discrimination on the basis of race, color, or national origin in programs that receive federal assistance. Since almost all programs and institutions of higher learning utilize federal monies, they must comply with the law.

Another aspect controlled by federal funding is sex discrimination. Title IX of the Educational Amendments of 1972 prohibits discrimination against students on the basis of sex in programs or institutions receiving federal funds. This includes programs and activities in secondary education, and it specifically identifies the prohibition against sex discrimination in admission and grading and evaluation procedures in institutions of higher learning. Sex bias in nursing by health professionals has existed for many years. If this is a problem in a specific nursing program, immediate steps should be taken to eliminate the source or cause, and steps should be taken at once to rectify the situation.

Statements 8, 12, and 20 relate to curriculum development and the formulation of policies and procedures. In order to have student input into curriculum development and revisions, students should be included as active members of the policy and procedural committees. This supports student involvement in the educational process as well as providing opportunities for student learning. Contributions by the student in curriculum development can be invaluable and should be encouraged. Just as follow-up studies are a method of product evaluation, student participation in curriculum planning is a process evaluation of the program's curriculum. Student evaluation of curriculum, policies and procedures, courses, instructors, and grading methods is important to the growth process of the nursing program.

Expectations between students and nursing faculty are discussed as a student right in statement 13. The nurse educator must be responsible for informing the students of the institution's educational expectations. Initially the nurse educator should discuss with students the philosophy and conceptual framework of the program. This provides the foundation for the level, course, and classroom objectives as well as the evaluation methods. The syllabus for each class should be provided to the students with explanations about the course content, course units, and class objectives. Classroom evaluations (quizzes or tests) should be identified on the course syllabus according to class objectives.

In the clinical setting, the student should also be supplied with the clinical objectives and an explanation of how they tie in with the philosophy and conceptual framework of the program. Clinical evaluations should be discussed with all students receiving copies of performance criteria. If anecdotal notes are part of the evaluation, students should be told how to use them. Meeting with the student to discuss objectives and evaluation procedures is basic to any nursing program and should be viewed as a vital guide to mutual educator-student expectations and performance.

The Fourteenth Amendment to the Constitution of the United States guarantees the right to due process of law. In 1961 the U.S. Court of Appeals ruled that students also have this basic right of due process. The educational institution must provide the student with notification of grounds for any discipline, including dismissal, and provide a hearing for the student related to the disciplinary action. Statement 14 of the Student's Bill of Rights speaks to the issue of due process and affirms the educator's accountability in this procedure.

Statement 6 discusses the right to a procedure for grievance of suspected academic or disciplinary injustices. According to Logsdon et al., a procedure for student grievances serves several purposes:

1. It provides the student with recourse.
2. It affords the student the right to due process under the Fourteenth Amendment that is fair, equal, and reasonable treatment—without affecting the institution's right to administer an organized program of instruction.
3. It protects faculty rights to freedom of instruction.
4. If the student pursues the grievance outside of the institution in the civil court system, it provides data for the court to review and make a "due process ruling" without having to evaluate academic evidence.
5. It can mediate potential faculty abuse of power in academic evaluations by looking at the process of instruction (Were all students treated equally and fairly?) vs. the outcome of instruction (questioning faculty decisions in evaluation of specific content).[11]

A grievance procedure should be developed by both faculty and students and should provide the students with a mechanism of due process. Exhibit 3–9 is a sample grievance procedure.

Exhibit 3–9 Grievance Committee Procedure

The committee for reviewing student grievances should consist of the following individuals: 1 faculty representative and 1 student representative from each educational level. Should students, individually or as a group, believe that their rights, as outlined in the Student Bill of Rights, have been violated, the following procedure should be activated:

Step 1   The student or students claiming a violation of student rights will initially approach the individual or individuals involved and attempt resolution to the student's or students' satisfaction.

Step 2   After completing step 1, the student or students who are not satisfied with the results of the initial action will request a meeting of the Student Rights Committee. A written request must be submitted within one month of the alleged violation. Three days prior to the scheduled hearing, a written report of the student's/students' case must be submitted.

Step 3   The student or students will present the individual or joint case at the scheduled meeting and bring evidence that is pertinent to the issue. After hearing the case as presented by the student or students, the committee will make a judgment whether a hearing is warranted. A two-thirds vote is needed before the committee can act further in the student's or students' behalf. The student or students will be notified in writing of the committee's decision.

Step 4   Should the Student Rights Committee decide to represent the student or students, a meeting will be scheduled between committee members and the individual or individuals involved. The person or persons involved will receive ample notification prior to the meeting as well as a written copy of the problem. Each party in the violation will be asked to submit evidence and names of witnesses (if appropriate) five days prior to the hearing. The committee will exchange the written reports between parties.

Step 5   The representing Student Rights Committee members will meet and discuss the alleged violation of student rights with the person(s) involved. Each party will have an opportunity to present the case and to respond to the other party's presentation. The committee will then ask questions of either party for clarification. The committee will then deliberate and make a decision. Should the vote result in a tie, the chairperson or dean will be asked to cast the deciding vote. Tapes of the sessions will be provided to the chairperson or dean for this purpose.

Step 6   If the student, students, or faculty are dissatisfied with the results of this meeting, the committee will notify the individual(s) involved that further action is referred to the college or university grievance committee for further action.

Step 7   A written summary of the hearing with rationale for the decision will be sent to both parties and the chairperson or dean.

A crucial issue in education today is the student's right to educational privacy. Items 7 and 9 of the Student's Bill of Rights refer to student privacy with regard to records and files and the procedures for disclosure. A law that has influenced this right is the Buckley Amendment to the Family Educational Rights and Privacy Act of 1974. This law states that the student who is 18 years of age or the parent of said student who is under 18 years of age must have access to his or her record for the purposes of inspection and challenging. Further, the law states that no other party shall have access to the student's records without permission from the student and/ or the parent. Institutions that violate this law are penalized by the loss of any federal assistance that they receive.

According to Flygare, the following elements of this law are significant:

1. Students (or their parents) must be given access to their records within 45 days from the time a request is made.
2. Students (or their parents) must be granted a hearing by institution upon request to determine the validity of any document in the students' files.
3. Confidential letters or statements placed in the file prior to January 1, 1975, need not be disclosed under the law.
4. Students may waive their rights of access to confidential letters regarding admission, honors, or employment.
5. An educational institution cannot, with certain exceptions, release personally identifiable information about students.
6. Educational institutions must notify students and parents of their rights under the law.[12]

Source: © 1975, Phi Delta Kappa Educational Foundation. Reprinted with permission.

The law safeguarding student records' privacy is relevant to the nurse educator because of its ramifications in file keeping. Personal counseling files and health records should not be placed in a central file. Decentralization of pertinent material will prevent accidental access by individuals not directly involved with the contents. The educator should be aware that all students have the right to copy the material in their respective records and challenge the contents of those files. (A side benefit of this policy is that it eliminates collection of useless and irrelevant papers.)

A concern to nurse educators is who should have access to student records other than the students. Other educators within the nursing program should have access to the files for educational purposes. Administrators within the institution and accrediting agencies should also be provided use of the files for appropriate data. However, a log should be kept in each student's file of the individuals who have viewed the contents and the time and date of the action. A faculty-student conference would provide a basis for deciding which documents should be kept in each student's file as well as informing students about the law and their rights.

Student rights are as important to the nurse educator as they are to the nursing students. In order to function well within the educational setting, the clinical instructor must know students' legal rights. The foregoing should provide the nursing teacher with the background necessary for classroom teaching and clinical instruction.

CLINICAL INSTRUCTION

Accountability and clinical instruction must be centered around the legal and ethical aspects of nursing practice. In order for the nurse educator to be an effective clinical teacher, it is necessary to evaluate learning experiences according to quality, applicability, and accountability. This means that it is necessary to determine whether the experience provides good learning opportunities for the student, meets the course and clinical objectives, and embraces the legal and ethical standards for the practice of nursing.

Clinical instruction, whether it be for the student in a professional nursing school or for the graduate in an orientation program, involves accountability. Teachers must provide learners with optimum educational experiences within the framework of the health agency while maintaining safety standards of nursing care for clients. Learners must assume responsibility for their own educational goals and outcomes as well as for professional nursing competence. Clients have rights to professional nursing care provided by qualified individuals. Students who perform professional nursing acts during their clinical experience must complete them with the same degree of competence as any other professional nurse. This places a great deal of responsibility upon the instructor for selecting appropriate learning experiences within the realm of the experience and education of the student.

It is therefore imperative that the clinical instructor provide supervision for the student in situations where there is the slightest doubt of the student's abilities and competencies. Students must also assume responsibility for their actions and be encouraged to evaluate their abilities and competencies before performing a task for which they have not had experience or sufficient education. Accountability must be accepted by both teacher and learner in selecting the best learning experiences within safe limits of professional practice for the learner.

Since the head nurse and supervisor are ultimately responsible for client care, the hospital should have assurance from the educational institution that students (or graduates) are academically and clinically competent to provide professional nursing care. The Joint Commission on Accreditation of Hospitals (JCAH) has recommended that acknowledgment of this responsibility be incorporated into the contractual agreements between the institution and the cooperating health agency. A statement identifying the role of the head nurse and supervisor and client care might read as follows:

Contract Responsibility

The ultimate responsibility for client care rests with the health care agency. The agency's head nurse or designee will cooperate with faculty to meet the educational goals.

In order to maintain the competence of student nurses in clinical practice, clinical evaluations are performed periodically (see Chapter 11). Other methods of assuring the health agency of high-quality performance in clinical practice by the students and instructor would be to inform specified staff members of the course content, clinical objectives, evaluation procedures, and supervisory techniques used in the educational process.

Nursing Education and Client Rights

In the process of clinical instruction, conflicts often occur between nursing practice, medical practice, and the client's rights. The conflicts between nursing and medicine usually arise because of a risk-taking situation, where *risk-taking* is defined as an activity that involves a varying degree of perceived or real physical danger.

The AHA Patient's Bill of Rights supports the client's right to receive information about his or her diagnosis, prognosis, and treatment. Each client has the right to enough information to give informed consent and the right to receive instructions about treatment and health care. Informed consent is a considerable issue in nursing because of its implication to the professional nurse and its importance to the well-being of the client. Informed consent means that the physician must share with the client all information about a proposed treatment or therapy that the client needs in order to make an intelligent decision. This definition excludes the nurse from liability for providing an explanation of the medical care to the client. Although often nurses are asked to witness a client's signature on the form, it does not mean that they should be held accountable for disclosure of specified information. The nurse is giving witness to the client's signature on the form, not to the client's knowledge about the treatment or therapy. Thus the duty of witnessing a signature does not actually fall within the realm of professional nursing.

Since providing the information to the client about therapy or witnessing the signature is not within the domain of the professional nurse, then what role does the professional nurse have with regard to informed consent? The main responsibility of the nurse is to inform the physician either of the client's oral withdrawal from the consent should there be a change of heart or of the client's apparent lack of information concerning the treatment or therapy. Since oral withdrawal from the contract is binding, it is essential that the nurse be aware of the client's decision and expressed desire to stop the procedure. Nurses should be alert to questions from clients concerning what is going to happen, the risks involved, and the possible outcomes.

Should a student become involved in a client's withdrawal of consent or lack of knowledge, again the instructor should encourage the student to participate in solving the problem but should not insist on action, because action would mean high-risk confrontation. The student should report to the head nurse and notify the physician of the client's withdrawal of consent or lack of knowledge concerning the procedure. The student should immediately document the client's actions and the physician's response on the medical record. In cases where there might be legal problems, it would be best if the instructor cosigned this documentation. After the student has reported the entire incident to the head nurse and supervisor, the situation is within the hands of the health agency, where it presumably will be dealt with by appropriate personnel.

Most nurse practice acts identify health teaching of the client as an important aspect of professional nursing practice. However, there are still physicians practicing medicine who withhold information from their clients about tests, treatment, medications, blood pressure, and so on. Another concern expressed by many physicians has to do with the client's response to knowing about the side effect of drugs: "Clients who know about side effects are sure to have them." If this is the attitude of physicians about the client's ability to deal with information, what does it say about the physician? What does it say about the professional nurses who comply with the wishes of such a physician? Since the duty to inform the client is included in most registration laws, professional nurses are held legally responsible for supplying this information to the client. The student should be instructed to share all possible information with clients, from what medication has been prescribed to the specific plan for nursing care. Physicians who find it difficult to accept this approach to health care should be consulted about their concerns. The nurse educator should discuss this issue with the physician in an effort to resolve any existing conflict concerning care given to the client.

Another aspect of the Patient's Bill of Rights that is supported by the PNA Consumer's Rights to Nursing Care is the client's right to refuse treatment. The professional nurse must support the client in this decision, which often leads to confrontation with other health team members. To a student this can be a very difficult and devastating experience without the assistance and direction of the nurse educator. It is sometimes easier for the instructor to assume the role of client's advocate rather than the student. Thus students have an opportunity to observe interactions at a safe distance while getting an idea of how to handle themselves in high-risk situations. After conflicts are over, instructors should sit down with students and discuss what happened. Role playing by students will help them to deal with the next situation involving risk-taking and conflict.

An important aspect of clinical instruction is the conflict between maintaining the client's rights and providing learning experiences for the students. By virtue of their dependent role in the health care system, clients often consent to care, treatment, and exposure that they normally would reject. Instructors may seek approval from clients prior to using them in nursing rounds, client conferences, or group observations, but what choice do the clients have to say no? They are coerced into the situation because they believe that the quality of health care they will receive depends upon their compliance. Both students and nurse educators should be alert to signals from clients that all is not well, that while verbally saying Yes, nonverbally a client may be saying No.

Several steps can be taken to prevent violation of the client's right to privacy. The nurse educator should sincerely evaluate the need for group conference and nursing rounds as a method of clinical teaching. Other strategies can be as effective but protect the client's privacy. Multiple assignments should be used only as a last resort for good learning opportunities. Although the literature reports that this is an effective teaching method, the validity of such a strategy should be questioned when considering the client's rights. Students should be accountable for their own clinical assignments and not be reassigned for educational purposes (checking the decubiti on a client not assigned). The nurse educator should limit group care by the students and use more than one student for care of a client only when absolutely necessary. A rights statement like the following can be adopted by a nursing faculty to safeguard the rights of clients cared for by students in the nursing program:

Human Rights Statement

No student, other than the assigned student for that client, except when additional assistance is needed, will be allowed to observe a client, procedures, and/or equipment.

Such a statement limits to some degree the learning opportunities of the nursing students. Despite the limitation, however, this does not mean that students receive poorer clinical experience. It just means that the nurse educator must be a little more creative and work a little harder to find valuable clinical experiences for the student while still protecting the rights of the client. Although very few legal precedents have been set on the subject of liability in nursing education, it seems to be generally agreed that a student committing a negligent act is held liable for his or her actions, as is the instructor and all members in the chain of authority in both the health agency and the institution of higher learning. Faculty should be aware that if a student has had instruction and supervision in a particular skill, this student can be passed as having achieved mastery. If an error subsequently results because of the student's misperforming the supposedly mastered skill, the faculty's liability is reduced. Consider for example the case of the senior student who has successfully completed classes on medications and their administration and has had repeated supervised experiences. If this student administers a drug to the wrong client because of failure to follow correctly the procedure for identifying the client, the burden of liability rests with the student, not the faculty.

Student Liability

Faculty should create an atmosphere whereby students feel free to ask questions. If freedom to question is not felt, serious errors can result. It is important for all professional nurses to carry malpractice insurance. Those who do not, do so at their own risk. Not only should nurse educators and nursing students carry insurance because of the danger of error in judgment and practice, but it behooves all professional nurses to do so as well. Many hospitals and institutions hold policies that cover their employees, but many do not. Before one assumes that one is covered by such a policy, one should read the document very carefully. Even the best blanket coverage policy held by an institution does not usually supply the professional nurse with enough coverage in case of litigation.

If the student or graduate commits an act of negligence, the error should be reported, charted, and appropriate action taken. The student should report the occurrence to the head nurse (and anyone else designated by the head nurse) and notify the physician of the incident. This is sometimes done by the head nurse and should be left up to his or her discretion. The entire sequence of events should be charted on the client's medical record, including the course of treatment ordered by the physician. The student should also fill out the appropriate health agency incident report with the cooperation of the supervising instructor. The report is then kept on file by the health agency for future reference.

The educational institution should have its own report of the incident; many schools use a form similar to the ones used by health agencies (see Exhibit 3–10). The form should be completed by the student involved and contain details of the incident. The instructor should also submit a report relating the negligent act. Who handles this type of situation in a nursing program will depend upon the structure of the school. Usually someone in authority in the nursing program discusses the incident with both the student and the instructor and suggests the best way to handle the situation.

No error in judgment, no matter how minor, should be considered trivial. If students are to learn accountability, they must learn to act responsibly. They should be confronted with any negligent acts and made to account for their actions. On the other hand, once an incident is over, no "big deal" should be made of it. Wringing hands and moaning will not undo what the student has done or failed to do. Since each incident should be handled individually and there is no stock response to this situation, the report of the incident should be kept in the student's file until graduation, and then discarded. This provides a basis for establishing a pattern of behavior if the student performs more than one act of negligence.

Exhibit 3–10 Incident Report Form

An *incident* is any happening that is not consistent with the educational practices of the nursing program or one in which the safety of the client is jeopardized. It may involve an act of commission or omission.

Date of incident _____   Student involved _____

Level of student _____

DESCRIPTION OF INCIDENT—By the student

Signature _____

(Student)

DESCRIPTION OF INCIDENT—By the educator

Signature _____

(Educator)

OUTCOME OF INCIDENT

REPORT OF STUDENT CONFERENCE   Date _____

SUMMARY

Clinical instruction involves accountability to the student, consumer, agency, and institution of higher learning. Each instructor is accountable to the students to provide the best possible learning experience but is also responsible to the clients and cooperating health agencies. They must be aware of their role in the clinical setting and acknowledge the role of the agency in cooperation with that of the educational institution. Students must also be held accountable for knowing their individual abilities and limitations in providing health care within the scope of professional nursing practice. They too must be responsible to consumers to provide the best possible care and to health agencies to practice within the rules and regulations governing the joint contractual agreement.

Accountability and nursing are inseparable. As members of the health professions, professional nurses are responsible to the consumer for health care and to the state board of nursing examiners for competent care. The nurse is accountable first to the consumer, next to the profession of nursing, and last to the employing institution. Unfortunately, this order is sometimes reversed. Thus, nurses must continue to accept the challenge of accountability as health care needs of the consumer change. It is the responsibility of every professional nurse to acknowledge his or her obligations to self, the nursing profession, and society.

NOTES

1. *Webster's Third New International Dictionary, Unabridged* (Springfield, Mass.: Merriam-Webster, 1961).

2. Victor Robinson, *White Caps: The Story of Nursing* (Philadelphia: J.B. Lippincott, 1946), 282–283.

3. Milton J. Lesnik and Bernice E. Anderson, *Nursing Practice and the Law* (Philadelphia: J.B. Lippincott, 1947), 306–307.

4. Ibid., 316.

5. "American Nurses' Association Board Approves a Definition of Nursing Practice," *American Journal of Nursing* 55 (December 1955): 1474.

6. American Nurses' Association, *Memo to Executive Director of State Nurse's Associations and State Boards of Nursing* (Kansas City, Mo.: ANA, April 3, 1970).

7. State of Washington Nurse Practice Act, Title 18, Section 18, 88.050, 1973.

8. New York State Education Law, Title 8, Article 139, 6902, 1972.

9. State of Washington Nurse Practice Act.

10. Dorothy Mereness, "Freedom and Responsibility for Nursing Students," *American Journal of Nursing* 67 (January 1967): 69–71.

11. Jann B. Logsdon, Patricia K. Lacefield, and Mary Jo Clark, "The Development of an Academic Grievance Procedure," *Nursing Outlook* 27 (March 1979): 184–190.

12. Thomas J. Flygare, *The Legal Rights of Students* (Bloomington, Ind.: The Phi Delta Kappa Educational Foundation, 1975). © 1975, Phi Delta Kappa Foundation.

SUGGESTED READINGS

Besh, Linda Briggs. "Informed Consent: A Patient's Rights." *Nursing Outlook* 27 (January 1979): 32–35.

Christman, Luther. "Accountability and Autonomy Are More Than Rhetoric." *Nurse Educator* 3 (July/August 1978): 3–6.

Creighton, Helen. *Law Every Nurse Should Know*. Philadelphia: W.B. Saunders, 1975.

———. "Qualifications of Nursing Students." *Supervisor Nurse* 4 (February 1973): 51–53.

Kelly, Kathleen, and Eleanor McClelland. "Signed Consent: Protection or Constraint?" *Nursing Outlook* 27 (January 1979): 40–42.

McMullan, Dorothy. "Accountability and Nursing Education." *Nursing Outlook* 23 (August 1975): 501–503.

Millard, Richard M. "The New Accountability." *Nursing Outlook* 23 (August 1975): 496–500.

National League for Nursing (ed.). *Accountability: Accepting the Challenge*, Pub. no. 16-1621. New York: NLN, 1976.

———. *Accountability: A Challenge to Educators*, Pub. no. 16-1594. New York: NLN, 1975.

———. *Accountability: The Obligation of the Educational Institution to the Consumer*, Pub. no. 23-1690. New York: NLN, 1977.

———. *Instructor Accountability: Issues, Facts, Impact*, Pub. no. 16-1626. New York: NLN, 1976.

Chapter 4

Creativity: A Method of Instruction

Creativity in nursing is a relatively new subject under consideration. Traditional practices and experiences have closed the minds of nurse practitioners, nurse educators, and nurse researchers to the role of creativity in nursing. Much is being written about creativity even though there is a great deal yet to be learned. Before creativity can be applied to nursing, it must be viewed in its purest sense. This removes creativity from practice and sets it up for review as a philosophical concept.

CREATIVITY

Creativity has long been studied in the attempt to identify its source and its development. Theories of creativity have ranged from belief in mystical endowment of skills to belief in an inherent quality existing at birth. Individuals exhibiting certain behaviors were described as creative and given such labels as "artist," "inventor." Anyone not identified as having this supposed innate ability was not expected to produce creatively.

More recently, investigations have been directed toward discovering whether creativity can be developed through a learning process and thus be teachable. Based on a 1972 survey in which they conducted 142 experiments concerned with the teachability of creativity, Torrance and Torrance concluded that creativity was indeed teachable and that creative behavior could be developed through a teaching and learning process.[1]

To impart creativity through an organized method of instruction, the educator must view creativity as present in all individuals. Although creativity is no longer viewed as a "God-given trait" exhibited by only a select few, the extent of innate creativity may differ to some degree from person to person. It continues to be demonstrated in varying amounts, because of differences in individual talents and pursuits and stimulation of creative potential. Creativity is built upon a person's perceptions, feelings, and past experiences. Thus, the degree of each person's creativity depends not only on individuality and the desire and ability to create, but also on the promotion of that desire and abilities by creative instruction.[2]

Creativity is the process that is used to produce a new idea, thought, concept, or object. It is a deliberate act of inquiry that results in a product that need only be new to be deemed creative. Likewise, the value of the product is judged by the creative person and must be satisfying and meaningful to the self.

Creativity in this context is a quality that exists in each individual and can be demonstrated under appropriate circumstances. Choosing to be creative is necessary for the activity to take place. This concept of creativity is often very difficult for individuals to understand since they are often tied to the old belief system, that is, that creativity is an innate quality exhibited only in a select group of persons. Nursing must discard this concept of creativity and realize that it is a learned activity that can be nurtured to a high level in interested persons.

CREATIVITY IN NURSING

Creativity is a very important part of the problem-solving process. It provides a foundation for seeking alternatives when problems arise for which no immediate solution can be identified. Nurses have to recognize their creative potential and proceed to exhibit creativity in their practice. Steele and Maraviglia have identified a representative list of variables that influence the existence of creativity in nursing. These include:

1) Nurses must value creativity as important to the profession.
2) Environments where nurses perform must allow the freedom necessary for creativity to emerge.
3) Rewards for performance must reflect an awareness of the value of creative pursuits.
4) Educational programs for preparing nurses must allow opportunities for developing creative potential.
5) A reawakening and emphasis on the humane aspects of nursing are essential.
6) Client-centered nursing practice must continue to replace functional structured nursing practice.
7) Flexibility in thought and action must be the building blocks for the profession.
8) Autocratic climates must be replaced with democratic climates.
9) Nurses must be supportive of one another's achievements in order to stimulate continual creative activities.

10) Nurses must possess the self-confidence to become risk-takers.
11) Nurses must have a personal as well as a professional commitment to the advancement of the profession.[3]

Nurses should evaluate their own practice to determine the creativeness of their interventions and identify areas where creativity should be used.

Nurses identify the nursing process as the basis for all nursing interventions but often do not realize that the nursing process is a modification of the problem-solving process. Thus, in order for the nursing process to be used effectively, it is imperative that nurses recognize the role of creativity in this process.

Creative Problem Solving

Creative problem solving is used when a problem is unclear or no solutions to the problem are evident. It is effective because it taps resources that the nurse did not know existed. It motivates the user toward inquiry and freedom of choice and helps the individual reach outside the bounds of known nursing principles for imaginative applications of nursing interventions.

There are four steps in the creative problem-solving process: (1) data collection, (2) problem identification, (3) alternatives selection, and (4) solution evaluation. Obviously, similarities can be discovered between this process and any form of decision making. What is unique about this process is not the steps, but the way each step is activated.

During the first stage of the process, data collection, the problem solver gathers all pertinent information about the question or problem. In collecting the data, six all-important questions should be raised: What? Where? When? How? Who? and Why?

- *What* do I want to know about the situation? What information should I gather? What is the problem?
- *Where* do I get the information I need? Where does the problem occur?
- *When* does the problem occur? When does the problem seem more evident?
- *How* can I gather more information about the situation? How could it be different?
- *Who* is involved in the situation? Who should be consulted about information?
- *Why* is this a problem?

Such information gathering will help clarify the situation so that the process will automatically lead to the second step, problem identification.

Since problems related to providing appropriate nursing care are not always specific and clear-cut, the problem should be restated at least ten different ways at this stage. The problem may be broadened or made more specific according to the situation. Creative problem solving is many times more effective if it involves group participation. Thus, the nurse may wish to bring the problem before a group of nurses in a unit conference or proceed with the process on an individual basis. After the problem has been restated numerous times, the nurse or group must select the one statement that best typifies the problem. This statement will then become the definition of the problem.

The problem solvers must now think of alternatives for solving the problem stated. Suggesting all possible solutions is called *brainstorming*. In brainstorming a group produces ideas without judging the quality of the suggestions. It is important for all members of the group to defer judgment of any ideas generated during the session; all ideas must be accepted by the group as possible solutions to the problem.

After a list of alternatives for solving the problem has been developed, they are evaluated to determine their feasibility. Each solution is evaluated and alternatives to it are then listed in the same manner as the first time. Modifications and combinations of solutions can be made during this step, as many of the outlandish ideas are brought into perspective. The individual or group must now select the most reasonable solutions and evaluate their feasibility.

The criteria frequently used to determine applicability include: effect on the client or student, desires of the client or student, rules and regulations of the institution, time, and availability. Each situation and problem would require the students to develop a set of applicable criteria. A simple rating scale of good, average, and poor may be used also to evaluate each alternative.

Consider the following example:

> *Data collection.* Ms. Grey is 68 years of age. She is recovering from a stroke and has progressed well. Her speech is not noticeably affected, but her right arm, hand, and fingers are immobile. She is to be encouraged to exercise her entire body and is trying to do this, but she finds exercising her body and limbs a tiring experience and will only do it under direct supervision. She carries her right arm and hand around as she walks and she walks with a slight limp in her right leg, but manages without mechanical assistance.

> *Problem identification.*
>
> 1. How can Ms. Grey be encouraged to exercise more?
> 2. How can Ms. Grey walk more?
> 3. How can I convince Ms. Grey that her exercises are good for her?

4. How can I make Ms. Grey enjoy exercising?
5. How can Ms. Grey use her arms, hands, and fingers more?
6. How can Ms. Grey be made to understand the importance of exercising?
7. How can Ms. Grey recuperate faster?
8. How can I assist Ms. Grey in her exercises?

After listing the problems and all possibilities, the one that seems the most appropriate is selected and modified as necessary. Problem 5 seems to be the one that would help Ms. Grey the most. Modification of this statement might be

"How can I make Ms. Grey enjoy"
1. Exercising fingers
2. Exercising hands and arms
3. Exercising legs
4. Exercising entire body

After selecting items 1 and 2, the next step of the process can be applied accordingly.

Selecting alternative solutions. After the exact problem has been selected for appropriateness, alternatives must be provided for solution. This is done through free thinking and brainstorming, while deferring judgment.
1. Do finger exercises
2. Use model clay
3. Squeeze a rubber ball
4. Sculpt
5. Finger paint
6. Knead bread dough

Evaluating the solution. Using the criteria of desirability by Ms. Grey, cost, availability, and practicability, the solutions are evaluated. Accordingly, solutions 2, 4, and 6 are ranked highest. However, Ms. Grey ranked 6 the lowest, and 4 was very low due to cost. Solution 3 ranked consistently moderate to high according to all criteria and was selected for the nursing intervention. This was only one aspect of her exercise need and creative problem solving could be used for determining care in the other areas listed.

This method of planning nursing care involves both the client and the nurse in creative problem solving. The results are extremely effective because of the input from both nursing and the client. Creative nursing care should be encouraged whenever possible and particularly when the exact problem is not known or readily identifiable.

Creativity can be learned, and creative problem solving can be taught. The nurse who recognizes the value of the process will convey its importance to other members of the health team in providing high-quality nursing care.

CREATIVITY IN NURSING EDUCATION

Creativity should be encouraged in all areas of nursing education. The nurse educator should apply the principles of creativity to both classroom and clinical instruction. Creativity in nursing education involves active participation by the student and instructor. The student has a responsibility to engage in active learning and the educator has a responsibility to provide an educational climate conducive to creative learning.

Nurse Educator

In order to provide optimal learning experiences and promote high educational standards, the creative teacher must demonstrate certain qualities in nursing practice.

1. Self-assertion through self-actualization
2. Internalization of a conceptual framework based on a nursing model
3. Knowledge of subject matter
4. Demonstration of clinical expertise
5. Demonstration of flexibility
6. Exhibition of leadership abilities

Self-assertion through Self-actualization

Basic to all assertive behavior is a sense of worth and dignity that results only from a positive self-concept and high self-esteem. Self-concept entails a view of the self through the eyes of another. That is, we see ourselves as we believe others see us. This opinion of self can be either positive or negative, depending on what inferences one has drawn from interpersonal relationships in past experience. Since self-concept is the basic attitude that one holds concerning oneself, it is the foundation of a person's relationship to self and others. All creative feelings and thoughts are wrapped up in the total view that individuals have of themselves. The individual who has a positive self-view will be better able to apply energy toward creative endeavors.

Self-esteem is also involved in self-awareness and behavior toward self and others. Self-esteem, very simply, is how one feels about oneself. Self-esteem is based on individual self-concept and can be either high or low. With high self-esteem, the individual's potential is increased and steps can be taken toward achievement of established goals. When a person is in a period of low self-esteem, accomplishment of goals is delayed for lack of initiative and motivation and creativity is stifled. Positive self-concept and high self-esteem are essential for self-actualization and ultimately then for self-assertion.

Part of the process of developing a positive self-concept and high self-esteem is identification of strengths and weaknesses. Knowing one's limitations will help the individual to maximize personal capabilities and channel behavior and potentialities in creative directions. Having achieved mastery of the self, one can then begin to behave assertively when dealing with others. (See Chapter 9 for references on assertive behavior.)

Internalization of a Conceptual Framework Based on a Nursing Model

The first step in creative teaching is to demonstrate the nursing model in nursing practice. Many nurse educators, while subscribing to the nursing model in the clinical setting, are very dependent. Their activities are usually physician-centered and they find it difficult to provide nursing care without a medical diagnosis and a physician's orders. Teachers who are primarily concerned with the medical aspects of the client-nurse interaction have obviously not given priority to the role of professional nurse. The nursing instructor must view the client as a unified whole, not as an illness or a pathophysiological condition, relying on nursing skills, not just on the physician's orders. The nurse educator who cannot function independently in nursing practice has not internalized the conceptual framework of a nursing program that is based on a nursing model.

A nursing model must first be understood and then internalized by the nursing instructor before it can be used to promote independent, creative nursing in others. Compliance without internalization will only impede the learning process. Most nurses who view nursing as a profession separate from the medical profession can see the logical necessity for a nursing model. Appropriate inservice education related to the nursing model can, it is hoped, make the importance of this framework clear and concise. Nurses must establish the priority of a nursing model in their own practice before the internalization process can be completed.

Exhibition of Knowledge of Subject Matter

To say that the nurse educator must have knowledge of the subject matter seems obvious and unnecessary. However, in emphasizing its importance in creative teaching and learning, knowledge has to be mentioned as a vital component of the teacher's qualifications. The teacher must know the material but must also be able to say "I don't know." In the educational setting, teachers should be assigned to the nursing course or clinical area in which they have had nursing education. Care should be given to avoid assigning faculty to subject areas that are unfamiliar. The educational program cannot expect all faculty to be experts in all subjects related to nursing and in all clinical settings.

Teachers in a hospital use the experts as resource persons. For example, a head nurse might see a need for special instruction to be provided to the staff or to one of the clients. A clinical specialist might be asked for special guidance, and so too could the inservice teacher. The nursing staff should use the expertise provided by the inservice teacher whenever appropriate.

All nursing educators, whether in hospitals, community health care, or educational programs, must be cautioned, however, as to whom to ask to be resource persons. If the nursing model has been internalized and is being taught, the medical staff must not be involved in the educational process except for the interpretation of medical orders. Just as it would be inappropriate for the nurse educator to teach medical students about medicine, it is inappropriate for the physician to teach nursing students about nursing.

Demonstration of Clinical Expertise

The clinical teacher has always been held in high esteem by others in the health professions. Often this esteem has not been earned but is based on the number of academic degrees after a name. For years clinical competence and nursing expertise were not considered criteria for employing individuals as nurse educators. Today, however, more and more requirements must be met in order for a person to be qualified to teach in a nursing program connected with an institution of higher learning. This change in employment standards has provided more competent nursing teachers and has improved the quality of nursing education.

 Clinical instruction is the teaching of nursing interventions based on theoretical knowledge and clinical skills. The clinical instructor who lacks appropriate nursing skills for nursing intervention is in a very risky position. In order to perform in situations that are life-threatening for the client and function as a role model to the nursing student, the nursing teacher should have developed above-average nursing competencies. A nursing educator lacking competencies may jeopardize the health and well-being of the client as well as hinder the education of the students. This is not to say that all instructors must display clinical expertise in all settings at all times. That would be unrealistic. It is realistic, however, to believe that all clinical instructors should have sufficient nursing competencies to function well within the standards of nursing practice. If this were true, then the old adage "Those who can do, do; and those who cannot, teach" could not be applied to nurse educators.

Demonstration of Flexibility

One essential quality of the creative nursing teacher is the ability to be flexible and open-minded. Flexibility means displaying an easygoing manner so that objectives and goals can be accomplished without imposing a forced structure. Flexibility encourages questioning—questioning not only of subject material, but also of techniques, methods, and procedures. Flexibility and open-mindedness are qualities that result from having a positive self-concept, high self-esteem, having internalized the conceptual framework, knowing the subject matter, and having clinical competence and expertise. Feeling secure in these areas, the nurse teacher will not be threatened by the lack of structure in the clinical situation.

For years rigidity in nursing has been its worst enemy. Priorities have included clean white uniforms and shoes; short, off-the-collar hair; tightly drawn sheets on beds; meeting the needs of the doctor; cleaning bedpans; and many other "important" aspects of nursing. What happened to the client? Has our preoccupation with appearances and tasks made caring for the client incidental and perhaps an annoyance? In order for the teacher to be flexible and open-minded in nursing, a great deal of soul-searching must be done. Such questions must be asked as Does it really matter if the nurse does not wear a cap? If the nurse wears a flower? If the bed is altered to please the client? If the client's bath is taken in the evening? And if the doctor has to find his or her own charts? More important questions must be answered such as Is the client assessment complete? Does the client understand the health teaching? Is the nursing care plan complete? Are the client goals realistic? and Have the nursing orders been carried out? Once nurse teachers evaluate their own priorities regarding nursing, they can begin to teach nursing care to students with the flexibility that is necessary for creative instruction.

Exhibition of Leadership Abilities

Contrary to most opinions, leadership is a learned ability. Since this ability is essential to creative teaching, the nurse teacher must learn leadership skills by acquiring certain behavior patterns. Characteristics of a good leader are based on the expectations of the group desiring to be led and therefore are concrete or abstract as the needs of the group demand. Leadership must be discussed in terms of skills rather than characteristics if behavioral outcomes are to be determined. Specific skills related to leadership include communication, group process, change theory, assertiveness, motivation, power versus authority, delegation of responsibility, decision making, and conflict resolution. The individual who has acquired these skills becomes adept in demonstrating the desired qualities of a leader. Chapter 10 will discuss leadership skills in more detail.

Creative nursing instructors function as leaders and change agents in the nursing profession. They are self-assured, self-assertive, and self-actualizing, and demonstrate how the theoretical foundation—the nursing model—is put into practice. Without a strong commitment to nursing and its future on the part of nurse educators, the nursing profession will be lost to physicians and the paraprofessionals. It is the responsibility of all nursing faculty to strive for the betterment of nursing, nursing education, and self-education. They should be committed to enrichment through literature review and participation in professional workshops and conferences. Each educational institution should encourage its faculty members to keep abreast of current clinical practices related to nursing and to attend academic or inservice courses to increase their knowledge related to teaching and clinical instruction. Regardless of the method, nursing educators must assume responsibility for updating their theoretical base and improving their clinical competencies.

Creative nurse educators fulfill their obligation to the students, who are the consumers of nursing education. They accept each learner as an individual with worth and dignity, recognizing the learner's need for self-actualization and personal growth within the nursing profession. The nurse teacher has the responsibility for selecting and organizing the learning experiences that are appropriate for specific course objectives. By providing educational opportunities, the educator stimulates, challenges, and guides the learner in the acquisition and application of scientific concepts and principles.

Nursing Students

Students or graduates enter the educational system with varied backgrounds that enhance or hinder their creative learning. Their intrinsic and extrinsic motives will influence how they perceive the cognitive process. Learners are sensing, thinking individuals who are responsible and goal-directed, each responding to the learning process according to differences that make the individual unique. A student's educational behavior is greatly influenced not only by the past, present, and expected future experiences, but also by individual motivation, desire, and effort to learn creatively.

Students who enter a nursing program should display certain behaviors that will assist them in the creative learning process and the successful completion of the educational program. Figure 4–1 depicts these behaviors.

Caring

The student must view the client as a person and demonstrate warmth and kindness in assisting the client with health care. Showing compassion in the client-nurse relationship is what we call *caring*. Caring occurs as the result of internalizing feelings of empathy or sympathy and tenderness. True caring occurs only when these feelings are actively displayed during nursing intervention. The

Figure 4–1 Essential Behavior for Creative Learning

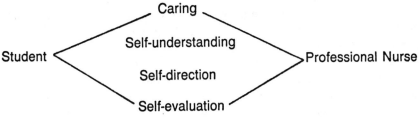

Student — Caring / Self-understanding / Self-direction / Self-evaluation — Professional Nurse

---

importance of this quality in a student of nursing cannot be stressed enough. Personal involvement means that the student is dealing with the client as a whole person rather than as an illness, a disease, or an educational experience.

Caring is a humanistic process that represents an emotional bond between individuals. For years nurses were educated to control their personal emotional involvement with clients and their families. This created the ''cold'' nurse and the ''superficial'' nurse who physically and mentally retreated from clients needing emotional support. Many educational programs still emphasize only the technical skills of nursing without due consideration of the personal commitment needed to provide total client care. Programs in nursing need to adopt caring as a concept within their conceptual framework in an effort to bring warmth, kindness, and compassion back into client care. This can be done without jeopardizing the emotional integrity of the student while still maintaining the supportive interaction with the client. The caring relationship between the client and the student evolves from more than just a concern for people; it must involve respect for individuals. Health agencies function to serve the needs of people, but the nursing profession functions to care for the needs of people.

Self-Understanding

It is vital that students be able to determine the ''why'' of their individual thoughts, actions, and feelings and then take appropriate steps in the management of their nursing education. Self-understanding is a dynamic process in which the student must participate for therapeutic use of self to occur. Self-understanding means getting to know oneself, becoming aware of all the thoughts, feelings, and behaviors that one experiences in dealing with self and others.

Students entering the nursing program often experience personal concerns about themselves and nursing. Fears and anxieties may block the learning process as great amounts of time and energy are spent on dealing with stress. This type of crisis occurs quite frequently and can incapacitate the nursing student and hinder learning. The nursing student can be helped through this situation by the creative nurse educator who is alert to the problem and responds appropriately by providing personal counseling. Once the source of the student's fears and anxieties is identified, steps can be taken to alleviate them through the appropriate coping mechanisms. It is only after this self-understanding occurs that the student will be able to achieve in the educational process.

Self-understanding not only assists students in dealing with their own goals and educational objectives, but also helps them work more effectively with others. As students gain knowledge about their own thoughts and actions, they will be able to understand more about the concerns and behavior of their assigned clients. This will, in turn, enable them to use their individual personalities as an effective nursing tool. Self-understanding can help the student to grow personally and professionally into a responsible, caring nurse.

Self-Direction

Students must be motivated to learn and to take the initiative in establishing their own educational goals. Motivation that comes from within the student is called self-direction and is a quality vital for the student's successful completion of the nursing program. Self-direction emphasizes individual learning and requires that the student spend a great deal of time and effort involved in learning. As sensing, thinking individuals, students must be held accountable for learning or failing to learn. They must each accept the responsibility of their own education and seek assistance from appropriate persons when needed. Self-direction allows the student freedom of choice and promotes a sense of responsibility needed for the management of the consequences of one's decision making.

Self-direction can often be identified in the new nursing student by creative behavior related to inquiry. Questioning by the student, although often irritating to the insecure instructor, denotes an inquisitive mind that should be fertilized by creative teaching and cultivated by a creative educator. Self-direction, an important trait in a student, should be encouraged throughout the nursing program. Self-direction should not stop at the end of the educational program but should continue throughout life. The profession of nursing is committed to the promotion of continued education for nurses. As a nurse, one must assume this responsibility for continued learning and seek enrichment through intellectual stimulation and creative exploration.

Self-Evaluation

Students should be urged to evaluate their own progress throughout the nursing program. Self-evaluation is vital to learning. Students should be able to identify their own strengths and weaknesses, diagnose areas of difficulty in learning, and establish a basis for change in their individual behavior.

The attempt to evaluate the self objectively is often very difficult. It may promote unrealistic views of oneself. The good student, during self-evaluation, tends to underrate his or her abilities and progress in an educational program, whereas the poorer student often does the opposite. The nursing instructor should work with the student in setting attainable goals and should assist in the self-evaluation. The evaluation process will be discussed in more detail in Chapter 11.

Self-evaluation is a personal experience that is meaningful only when it assists the individual toward self-actualization. Through self-actualization the student will gain self-confidence and self-esteem. Self-evaluation and self-criticism are avenues for the development of a positive attitude toward change. Experience in self-evaluation will not only enable the student to function more effectively as a practitioner of nursing but will reward the student in his or her personal life.

The Learning Process

Learning can be defined as the addition of new knowledge and skills that result in mental activity and behavior change. Learning can be active or passive depending on the degree of student involvement. Passive learning occurs when the instructor spends most teaching time conveying information that the students are expected to internalize without active participation. Active learning occurs when students invest time and effort to acquire knowledge. Learning is enhanced by an educational climate that promotes creativity, exploration, and freedom for discovery. The teacher acts as a facilitator who leads and guides the student through the education experience and a resource person who provides additional information to students when it is needed. The teacher must decide who is primarily responsible for student learning: the student or the facilitator.

In order to promote creativity in nursing instruction, emphasis should be placed on self-teaching, self-understanding, and self-evaluation. Rogers' definition of learning summarizes the qualities needed by the student in order for learning to occur. He identifies five characteristics of successful learning: it requires personal involvement; must be pervasive, self-initiated, and evaluated by the learner, and in essence must be meaningful.[4] Active learning is a self-directed activity involving a personal commitment by the learner. It is meaningful only when it is evaluated by the learner as relevant and satisfying to the self. Creative instruction, then, must be directly related to learning.

As participants in the creative learning process, students have a direct responsibility for active learning. They must recognize their own self-worth and dignity while establishing their respective educational goals. Nursing students should be made aware of their responsibility to be creative in the learning process. All available opportunities should be utilized for furthering students' individual learning objectives.

Creative students demonstrate qualities of imagination, initiative, individualism, and inquiry. They should be self-directed and self-disciplined in learning and uninhibited in thinking.

Students should be encouraged to ask questions and make independent judgments based on their individual level of competence. Often students are stifled in their attempts at inquiry into the scientific explanations of cause and effect. One of the main reasons is the insecurity of the teacher in this realm of questioning. Teachers find it easier to instruct the student who accepts without question the dictum of nursing knowledge, but the student who passively receives information without inquiry will be less likely to perform well as a creative nurse.

The Learning Climate

The teacher can stimulate creative learning by providing a climate that is flexible, permissive, and free. Students should feel safe to disagree with the teacher without jeopardizing their positions in the nursing program. Too often teachers are threatened by the student who dissents and will make every effort to curb such inquisitive behavior. As a teacher one must feel secure enough in one's abilities, knowledge, and self-esteem to encourage such student behavior and to say, when appropriate, "I don't know!"

The teacher and student should also have established a meaningful relationship if creative learning is to exist. The teacher should be familiar with the student's nursing goals, personal objectives, and plan of action related to learning. Each student should be looked at separately and the strengths and weaknesses of each should be recognized. Only by identifying individual qualities of the students can the teacher assist them in the learning process and motivate them toward behavioral change. Mutual respect and understanding in the relationship between the student and instructor constitute a climate conducive to creative teaching and learning.

Cooperating agencies utilized by the educational program should be introduced to the concept that creativity is an integral part of the curriculum. Before the teacher enters the clinical setting with students, the staff should understand the application of creativity to clinical instruction and student learning. Behaviors typical of creativity should be discussed so that nursing management is aware of the expected behaviors of faculty and students in the clinical setting. By introducing the creative process and creative activities to the staff at this time many problems associated with educational priorities will be avoided. This will enable the staff nurses on the unit to understand why the instructor encourages the students to select their own clinical assignments, to establish their own educational goals, to feel free to question an established technique or procedure, and to engage in many other free-thinking activities. The flexibility of the educator in the clinical setting will also be better understood if the staff understands that this is part of the educational process according to the philosophy of the nursing program.

Blocks to Creativity in Nursing Education

Creativity in learning can be inhibited by three major factors: personal difficulties, social forces, and environmental influences. Personal difficulties, which affect the creative process, can arise within the teacher or learner. The teacher sacrifices creativity who, in order to cover the designated material, continually utilizes one teaching strategy without variation. Teachers who consistently "spoon-feed" students because the material should be easy for them limit the students' creativity and learning processes. Many times the teacher is expecting low-level educational behaviors from the students, such as memorization and recall of facts, rather than emphasizing application, analysis, and synthesis of nursing principles. Opportunities for creative learning can be enhanced by self-teaching, original work, and exploration.

Students who depend entirely upon lecture material, teacher-student interactions, and textbook material block their own learning powers. They place too much trust in the words of the instructor and may not learn to question. Students often rely on one source as a basis for learning. Teachers reinforce this by testing only from lecture notes and/or textbooks. Students must actively strive to broaden their horizons in nursing by engaging in creative inquiry.

Conformity and cultural pressures are the most common social forces inhibiting creative behavior. Teachers rarely vary their teaching strategies because lecturing is acceptable, and students find it easy to take notes. When a new teaching method is introduced in an educational setting, teachers may be evaluated on the basis of how "different" the method is from the "norm," rather than on its effectiveness in promoting behavioral change. Students also are under pressure from society and peers to conform to previously established standards. Society encourages conforming for the sake of conformity, without regard for individual differences and need. The creative teacher must overcome these pressures and provide optimal learning experiences for the students.

Those social forces that limit creativity of student and teacher alike are usually related to administrative policies. A very structured and rigid conceptual framework that adheres to a closely prescribed curriculum will stifle any creative person attempting to teach effectively. Classroom objectives should be designed to assist the student and teacher in the educational process. If they are so restrictive that students cannot discuss special topics of interest or related clinical experiences, they fail to serve their valuable purpose. Flexibility must be built into all teaching plans in order for creative learning to occur.

Many educators consider themselves as liberal in outlook. Rules and regulations that forbid the student to engage in dissension, inquiry, and discovery are lethal to creative teaching and learning. Both the students and teachers must use every possible measure to change binding attitudes, rules, and policies in order to promote freedom in learning.

CREATIVE INSTRUCTION

Creative classroom teaching must directly correlate with creative clinical instruction. It is impossible to expect the teacher and student to be creative in one aspect of nursing education while taking a traditional approach to learning in another. In relating teaching strategies to clinical instruction, consideration must be given to the methods that can be used most effectively in both educational settings.

The two most frequently used teaching strategies in nursing are lecture and demonstration. These are popular because a set amount of material can be covered without interruptions due to listeners' divergent thinking. Learning promoted by these teaching methods, however, is completely passive because they force the listener to absorb information through the senses without becoming actively involved.

Lecture

The lecture is a teaching method in which the instructor does all or most of the talking to present information to the students. This method does not promote active learning and creative exploration. There are appropriate times for it, however, although they are less infrequent than its use would indicate. Abuse of this method occurs when it is used exclusively without thought to what other strategies might meet a class's objectives more effectively.

Demonstration

Exhibition of an act with an explanation is called demonstration. The demonstration strategy is used frequently in teaching nursing because of its applicability to the mastery of nursing skills. According to Heidgerken the two main advantages of this technique are that it promotes careful observation by the student and it presents the material to the student in a concrete and explicit manner forcing the student to visualize the explanation as well as hear it.[5] Strict use of this method of instruction for teaching nursing techniques, however, promotes rote behavior on the part of the students. It inhibits creative exploration of different ways of providing nursing intervention and stifles the students' ability to inquire and discover. The nursing instructor must provide opportunities for students to develop their creative learning talent and assist them in seeking new avenues of learning.

Teaching in the classroom lends itself to specific instructional methods such as lecture and demonstration. Clinical instruction on the other hand requires less structured methods of teaching and relies heavily upon the creative ability and instructional expertise of the teacher. Creative teaching is utilizing the process of exploration to facilitate active learning. Exploration can be defined as creative attempts to seek answers to posed problems or questions. Explorative techniques open to discovery and inquiry include group discussion, role playing, nursing rounds, and game playing.

Discussion

Discussion is utilized when interaction between members of a group is desired. This method allows the students to interact with one another as well as with the teacher. The content is usually free flowing with minimal direction by the discussion leader. Discussion is the main teaching strategy used in clinical conferences and can be used effectively in creative clinical instruction. Group discussion should always be preceded by advance preparation on the part of the group members. In clinical instruction, clinical objectives serve the purpose to inform the students of the topic for discussion during the clinical conferences and provide guidelines for the students related to client care. Exhibit 4–1 is a sample of clinical objectives that can be used to outline the focus for pre- and post-conference.

The clinical focus as demonstrated by the objectives listed in the exhibit will provide the beginning student with a clearly defined area for preparation and practice. ''Pre-'' and ''post-conferences'' will be discussed in more detail in Chapter 5.

Exhibit 4–1 The Nurse, Client, and Family: Clinical Focus on Elimination Needs of the Client

1. Identify the client's elimination patterns.
2. Discuss with the client the importance of good elimination patterns.
3. Identify factors that influence the client's elimination patterns.
4. Identify any deviations from normal in the client's human responses to elimination needs.
5. Examine client's records regarding
   a. Urine.
   b. Stool.
   c. Pertinent x-ray studies.
   d. Endoscopy procedures.
6. Discuss with the client prescribed medication that may influence elimination patterns.
7. Obtain urine specimen from the client and complete a urine reduction.
8. Describe nursing responsibilities used in assisting the client with elimination needs.
9. Provide nursing intervention related to elimination needs of the client.

Simulation

Game playing or simulation as a creative teaching strategy should be used only in supplemental activities for the student. Frequently, during a specified clinical period, the students complete their assigned care and have accomplished their educational goals for the day. Unless reassigned to care for other clients, students often waste this time looking for activities to keep busy. One good way to make sure students use such moments for learning is to provide mental games that are fun, educational, and based on the clinical focus and course content. For example, students caring for families during the antepartal period might utilize the logic game shown in Exhibit 4–2 and word scramble shown in Exhibit 4–3 to reinforce what they have learned.

In order to complete the logic problem in Exhibit 4–2 successfully, students must have basic knowledge about antepartal problems. They must be familiar with relevant terminology and the more severe problems that can occur during pregnancy. This type of logic problem can be developed in any health area. (See Appendix 4–A at the end of this chapter for the solution.)

A word scramble can be developed for any phase of nursing and related information. Most students enjoy this game and will be able to apply their knowledge of the drugs to the list. This is a brief sample of the use of word scramble in gaming. (See Appendix 4–A at the end of this chapter for the solution.)

Exhibit 4–2 A Logic Problem

The following is a logic problem concerning mothers, their gestation, and their antepartal problems. The mothers' names are Mary, Janice, Betty, Ann, and Darlene. Their gestations are two months, three months, five months, eight months, and full term. Their problems are toxemia, nausea and vomiting, diabetes, frequency of urination, and backache.

Using the above information and the following statements, determine each mother's gestation and her problem:

1. Mary does not have toxemia or diabetes and neither does the woman who is full term.
2. Betty is not three months' or five months' pregnant and is not full term.
3. The woman who is full term is not Janice, nor does she have backache.
4. Ann is five months' pregnant and has no minor discomforts.
5. Ann and the woman who has toxemia are not full term.
6. Mary had nausea and vomiting two months ago, but has no symptoms of it since.
7. Janice and the woman who is eight months' pregnant do not have urinary frequency or backache.

Exhibit 4–3 Word Scramble: Drugs in Obstetrics

nicipot	gitna
aiivslrt	etorregat

Exhibits 4–2 and 4–3 were two examples of games that were developed by the authors of this book. More sophisticated and commercial games for use in nursing programs are available for purchase. However, the complexity or the sophistication of games and simulation provide only as much education to the students as they are willing to contribute. It is therefore recommended that this teaching strategy be used only in addition to the other previously described methods of instruction.

Role Playing

Role playing as a teaching strategy is very effective in promoting improved interpersonal relationships. Cooper defines role playing as "the spontaneous acting out of problems or situations to gain insight by placing oneself in the position (role) of another."[6] Students who participate in role playing take an active part in their learning process. A sense of warmth and trust must exist in the group in order for effective role playing to occur. Because the students are personally involved in the activity, they tend to concentrate more on the learning situation and remain attentive to the educational experience.

This technique can be used very creatively and effectively in pre- and post-conferences when discussing therapeutic approaches to client intervention. For example, the students could role play the approach to a client with a concern or problem about sexuality. This would allow the student a practice session before discussing the subject directly with the client. Any interpersonal relationship problem can be solved by the use of this teaching strategy, since the learners have the opportunity to try out certain communication techniques and skills. Other situations in which this could be used effectively would be in reducing student anxiety related to dealing with the nursing staff. For students having problems related to staff relations, this technique should allow a tryout before the actual interaction occurs.

Role playing can involve a few of the group or all of the members may participate. One method for using this technique is to have two or three students role play a situation while the rest of the group watches the interaction. After the session is over, the onlookers can offer suggestions for improvement or support in the manner in which the students used the exercise. Another way to use role playing is for the entire group to separate into small groups and role play the same situation. After the session is over, the students each report to the whole group their feelings and responses to the interaction. Role playing by a few or the entire group will promote understanding and provide better learning experiences for the students.

This technique can be used very effectively by the inservice educator in orienting new graduates to new services, units, and personnel. The anxious newcomer may need some direction in handling the new experiences. Role playing can provide this person with the opportunity to try several approaches to the situation and select the most appropriate. Staff nurses who are responsible for teaching clients or other staff members may find this technique useful as a warm-up to the real thing.

Nurses should be encouraged to use this very effective teaching tool to improve their skills in relating to others. Likewise, nurses can assist clients using role playing to help them through a variety of personal crises. A client may practice what to say to the doctor about wishing a consultation with another physician; a child may act out feelings about the hospital experience, or a terminally ill client may rehearse the discussion of important funeral arrangements with the family. Role playing is effective any time that the learner or client needs to work through a problem in dealing with others. (See Chapter 8 for more on role playing.)

Programmed Learning

Programmed learning promotes self-direction in students as they can work at their own pace and learn the material with minimal assistance from the instructor. However, independent study should never be substituted for teacher-directed learning. The nurse educator should be available to discuss the content with students and answer questions about the material.

Instruction Texts

One of the best methods of learning on an independent basis is through the use of programmed instruction texts. Material is presented to students in order to provide a basis for further learning of the process. Specific situations are identified to which students must respond. Depending upon the students' response, they are instructed to either review the content being taught or directed to continue on to the next situation. All independent study based programs stress the content aspect of the course with minimal practical application. However, many good texts contain a sufficient amount of practical material to make them beneficial for student learning.

Computer Assisted Instruction (CAI)

Another teaching method that is becoming more popular in schools of nursing, is computer assisted instruction. Commercially prepared programs in nursing areas are limited, at present, but some do exist in special areas of nursing care. The alternative to buying prepackaged programs is for faculty to develop their own computerized self-instructional modules. This allows the educator to have a teaching tool specifically designed to meet the needs of students. However, the development of such programs requires that nurse educators be knowledgeable in computer programming, or consult with a computer specialist for assistance. Computerized instructional materials are beneficial as teaching tools and should be considered when selecting appropriate teaching strategies. Once the program is developed and operational, students can learn the subject matter independently, providing release time for nursing instructors.

Audiovisuals

Films, filmstrips, slides, audiotapes, and videotapes can be used as a teaching strategy for independent study or as a class activity. As an independent study activity, audiovisuals should supplement classroom content, not replace it. Audiovisuals can be used very creatively to focus on a particular aspect of learning. However, overuse of this strategy can promote passive learning in the student resulting in a poor learning experience.

Current films can be used to emphasize theoretical content. However, classroom use should be augmented through the use of study guides. Nurse educators can develop appropriate study guides that direct the students toward specific content. The study guide should be distributed to the students in advance of the showing in order that they understand the focus of the learning experience. Exhibit 4–4 is an example of a study guide that could be used for the film *On Golden Pond*.

Exhibit 4–4 Study Guide for *On Golden Pond*

---

1. Identify developmental tasks, stages, and situations of individuals and the family.
2. Contrast the role of the family members and how they are influenced by environment.
3. Identify the methods that the individuals used to communicate:
   a. Love
   b. Anger
   c. Frustration
   d. Fear
4. What types of supportive communications did the wife and husband use for each other?
5. How did the communications reflect developmental levels? perceptions?

SUMMARY

Creativity is important to nursing education. Creative nursing education must be provided by educators who are totally committed to the belief that students are self-directing and responsible individuals. Creative instruction encourages freedom to explore and ultimately promotes the retention of the explored learning experience.

For the educational process to be an effective and creative learning experience, both the educator and the student must be active participants. The clinical instructor has the responsibility for personal development of the qualities necessary to facilitate creative learning. The student must be open to creativity during the educational experience while exhibiting the characteristics of a caring person.

The principles of creative teaching strategies must be considered prior to the selection of specific learning activities. Educators must incorporate creativity into all educational experiences in order to promote the qualities of self-direction and responsibility in the student. Creative teaching strategies enhance the educational experience of the student while relating the concepts of flexibility and openness to the practice of nursing.

NOTES

1. E. Paul Torrance and J. Pansy Torrance, *Is Creativity Teachable?* (Bloomington, Ind.: Phi Delta Kappa Educational Foundation, 1973), 2.

2. Ibid.

3. Shirley M. Steele and Frank L. Maraviglia, *Creativity in Nursing* (Thorofare, N.J.: Charles B. Slack, 1981), 62.

4. Carl R. Rogers, *Freedom to Learn*, ed. Carl R. Rogers and William R. Coulson (Columbus, Ohio: Bell and Howell, 1969).

5. Loretta E. Heidgerken, *Teaching and Learning in Schools of Nursing* (Philadelphia: J.B. Lippincott, 1965), 428.

6. Signe S. Cooper, "Methods of Teaching—Revisited; Roleplaying," *Journal of Continuing Education in Nursing* 11:36, 57–58, January/February 1980.

SUGGESTED READINGS

Bevis, Olivia E.M. *Curriculum Building in Nursing: A Process.* St. Louis: C.V. Mosby, 1978.

Clark, Carolyn Chambers. "Simulation Gaming: A New Teaching Strategy in Nursing Education." *Nurse Educator* (November/December 1976):4–9.

Cooper, Signe S. "Methods of Teaching—Revisited." *Journal of Continuing Education in Nursing* 9 (July/August 1978):24–25.

———. "Methods of Teaching—Revisited; Brainstorming." *Journal of Continuing Education in Nursing* 9 (November/December 1978):16–18.

———. "Methods of Teaching—Revisited; Games and Simulation." *Journal of Continuing Education in Nursing* 10 (September/October 1979):14, 47–48.

———. "Methods of Teaching—Revisited; Informal Discussion." *Journal of Continuing Education in Nursing* 9 (September/October 1978):14–16.

———. "Methods of Teaching—Revisited; Nursing Care Conference." *Journal of Continuing Education in Nursing* 10 (January/February 1979):28–30.

deTournay, Rheba. *Strategies for Teaching Nursing*. New York: John Wiley, 1971.

Hahn, Robert O. *Creative Teachers: Who Wants Them?* New York: John Wiley, 1973.

Holm, Karyn, et al. "A Teaching-Learning Experience: Nursing Rounds." *Journal of Nursing Education* 17 (April 1978):33–36.

Holt, John. *Freedom and Beyond*. New York: E.P. Dutton, 1972.

Kagan, Jerome (ed.). *Creativity and Learning*. Boston: Houghton Mifflin, 1967.

Layton, Janice. "Students Select Their Own Grades." *Nursing Outlook* 20 (May 1972):327–329.

Lowenfeld, Viktor, and W. Lambert Brittain. *Creative and Mental Growth*. New York: Macmillan, 1970.

Lundsteen, Sara W. "Questioning to Develop Creative Problem Solving." *Elementary English* 51 (May 1974):645–650.

Lytton, Hugh. *Creativity and Education*. New York: Schocken Books, 1972.

Massialas, Byron G., and Jack Zevin. *Creative Encounters in the Classroom: Teaching and Learning through Discovery*. New York: John Wiley, 1967.

Mereness, Dorothy. "Freedom and Responsibility for Nursing Students." *American Journal of Nursing* 67 (January 1967):69–71.

Michael, William B. (ed.). *Teaching for Creative Endeavor: Bold New Venture*. Bloomington, Ind.: Indiana University Press, 1968.

Miel, Alice (ed.). *Creativity in Teaching*. Belmont, Calif.: Wadsworth, 1961.

Ripple, Richard. "Communication, Education, and Creativity." *Contemporary Educational Psychology* 2 (1977):219–231.

Steele, Shirley, and Frank L. Maraviglia. *Creativity in Nursing*. Thorofare, N.J.: Charles B. Slack, 1981.

Taylor, Sandra, Mary S. Brodish, and Hazel N. Brown. "Creative Learning Experience for Student Nurses." *Journal of Nursing Education* 18, no. 4 (April 1979):16–18.

Thomas, Barbara. "Promoting Creativity in Nursing Education." *Nursing Research* 28, no. 2 (March-April 1979):115–119.

Appendix 4–A

Answer to Logic Problem in Exhibit 4–2

Name	Months	Complaint
Mary	3	Backache
Janice	2	Nausea and vomiting
Betty	8	Toxemia
Ann	5	Diabetes
Darlene	Full Term	Frequency

Answer to Word Scramble—Drugs in Obstetrics—in Exhibit 4–3

1. nicipot—PITOCIN
2. aiivslrt—VISTARIL
3. gitna—TIGAN
4. etorregat—ERGOTRATE

Chapter 5

Creative Clinical Instruction

Creative instruction is very applicable to all nursing educators whether they are instructors in nursing education or in inservice. The creative clinical teacher approaches each learning experience differently, seeing in each situation an opportunity for learning limited only by the needs and desires of the learner. It is essential to maximize every clinical learning experience by encouraging the learner to seek creative means to provide excellent nursing care.

NURSING EDUCATION

Clinical instruction is nontraditional education in a nontraditional setting. What occurs in this area is not dictated by standards established for classes held within the walls of institutions of higher learning. It is, in fact, a considerably more difficult type of teaching than classroom instruction. This is due partly to the nature of the location of the educational experience and partly to the lack of formal structure within which the educator must teach. For the same reasons many master's programs do not include courses on clinical teaching; this is a very problematic area for instruction. It is interesting to note that, despite the difficulty of this type of instruction, in the past most State Board of Nursing Examiners required only a bachelor's degree in nursing to engage in clinical instruction but a master's degree in nursing to teach in the classroom.

Such lack of emphasis on teaching clinical instruction, and on the importance of clinical instruction, promotes haphazard and coincidental learning during students' clinical experiences. In many schools of nursing, clinical instruction is not consistent from nursing course to nursing course, or from nurse educator to nurse educator. Such confusion occurs because nurse educators have not been taught to teach in the clinical setting. Oftentimes, they have only their own student experiences to guide them in their methods and strategies related to clinical instruction.

Clinical instruction has generally been synonymous with clinical supervision, that is, a "watching over" activity that served to protect the consumer from harm and provided the student with a resource for ensuring the safety of the client. As nursing education has become more sophisticated and quality oriented, clinical instruction has come to mean much more than the traditional act of directing care.

Nurse educators are now charged with the responsibility for establishing educational opportunities in the clinical setting that will result in a change in behavior of the learner. Although client safety is still of utmost importance, the focus in clinical instruction must also include learning experiences that expand students' nursing knowledge and promote growth in their professional lives.

This challenge for nurse educators means that more definitive questions about clinical instruction must be asked:

"What do I teach?"

"How do I teach?"

"What is needed to know?"

"What is nice to know?"

"Who is responsible when students learn?"

"Who is responsible when students do not learn?"

Although there are no specific answers to these questions, there are certain principles that should be addressed. For example, if selected assessment skills are identified as a "need to know" experience, each instructor has to assume responsibility for providing students with opportunities to acquire such skills. However, if the instructor has identified additional skills as "nice to know," time can be allotted for these experiences only if it does not sacrifice the learning of the "need to know" activities.

- *Students are in the clinical setting to learn professional nursing.*

This statement seems rhetorical and not applicable to clinical instruction. However, too many students are placed in clinical settings with no plan for learning. Clinical focuses and objectives should be used for the majority of clinical experiences. Chapter 6 discusses these learning tools.

Another problem often found in educating students in the clinical situation relates to the staff attitudes about the role of the student on the unit. In many institutions, students are considered the "extra help," the "go-fors," or the "clean-ups." Nurse educators fall into the compassion trap when they are asked such questions as "Mrs. Smith is ready to come back from Recovery. Do you have a student who is not doing anything?" "We are really busy, could your students help pass trays?" "The Laundry Room just called and has the linen ready. Do you have someone who can go get it?" "Boy, have we got a good client for you. Mr. Brown is on bed rest, has IVs, is semi-comatosed, needs a catheter inserted, and is partially incoherent. It would be a good experience for your students!'' Or "Since your students are just reading charts, maybe they could help clean up this unit. We have a client waiting downstairs for the bed.''

Nurse educators must be careful to keep in focus the reason for the learning experiences for the day. In their quest for "keeping the peace" with the staff, educators often permit and even encourage students to participate in these types of activities. Many times the staff needs to be reminded that the student has his or her assignment and that the clinical objectives for the day do not include these extraneous, nonprofessional activities. If problems continually arise in this area, the nurse educator should meet with the head nurse and staff to redefine the student's role on the unit.

- *Students learn best when classroom material is correlated with the clinical experience.*

One of the most difficult tasks for the nurse educator is to find the "right" type of client to assign students to during their clinical experience. If the classroom content addresses care of the client with a myocardial infarction, the nurse educator ideally should locate a client with this diagnosis for each of the students in the group. This is unrealistic in most cases. Such situations occur frequently, universally, and cannot be helped; thus, alternatives must be sought.

One way of ensuring a more uniform learning experience is to broaden the classroom content to include several acute heart problems, or broaden the clinical focus to encompass care of clients with various kinds of heart disease. If the classroom content is broadened, there are more opportunities for a larger variety of experiences in the clinical setting. However, if the classroom format is not flexible enough to provide for this change, the clinical focus can easily include many medical diagnoses that require similar nursing interventions. The most logical answer is to direct the clinical focus toward broad categories relating to client needs. Exhibit 5–1 provides an example of how a clinical focus can be adapted to account for the lack of specific medical diagnoses.

- *Clinical learning is directly related to the quality of clinical instruction provided.*

This statement identifies the need for good clinical instruction if maximum learning is to take place. It calls for educated teachers to clinically instruct students in a systematic and deliberate way. This means that instructors should always be available for students during the clinical experience. Instructors cannot effectively teach a large number of students; nor can they be available for assistance if students are assigned to clients in several clinical areas. The nurse educator should serve as a resource person, and in this role must be visible to the students at all times.

Exhibit 5–1 General Focus Sheet

FOCUS: Heart Disease

1. Assess the client with acute heart problems.
2. Discuss with the client his or her perceptions of the illness.
3. Review medical records as to abnormal reports.
4. Relate nutrition, activity, and life style to client's illness.
5. Establish with the client health goals related to the illness.
6. List nursing interventions specific to the client's illness.
7. Evaluate the plan of care with the client.

The nurse educator functions as a facilitator for learning. The students should have the opportunity to determine their own educational goals. In establishing these goals, learners should be given freedom of choice according to individual educational needs. They must each take the initiative in selecting learning opportunities that are satisfying as well as providing optimum learning experiences. Thus, learners assume responsibility for their own goals and the experiences that will help them meet their objectives. In this type of individualized learning, the nurse educator is the support for the students.

- *Clinical instruction should be creative.*

Creativity in nursing education should be encouraged in all aspects of the student's learning. If learning is to be successful, the nurse educator must establish creativity as a priority in clinical instruction. This means that the clinical instructor must have knowledge of creativity and its importance to quality nursing education and client care.

With the recent changes in the health care delivery system, fewer and fewer traditional clinical experiences are available for the nursing student. Nurse educators are forced to seek alternative clinical settings that provide similar educational experiences. In many cases, these alternative settings do not always provide for optimum learning for the nursing student. This places additional responsibility upon the nurse educator to either make the experience beneficial or find other clinical settings that provide maximum opportunities for learning.

Thus, in the process of providing quality education, the nurse educator must become creative in the selection of clinical experiences. Clinical instruction on specific units and in selected settings is not always feasible. Many times when it is, conditions are not optimal and the educator must break away from traditional methods and strategies of clinical instruction and creatively provide opportunities for nursing students that maximize their learning experiences and learning potential.

Creativity thus has a good deal to do with flexibility, openness, a willingness to adapt, experiment, and innovate. These values should be incorporated into every nurse's personal philosophy of nursing. If an educational program has encouraged creativity in the learning process and has promoted freedom for the exploration of alternatives for creative nursing care, the student will grow in creativity as a person and as a professional nurse.

INSERVICE EDUCATION

Like clinical instruction in a school of nursing, inservice education falls outside the realm of traditional classroom learning. At first glance, one might think that inservice education is a simple task, since the teacher has a "captive" audience. However, many problems arise because nursing does not place a high priority on learning experiences within the institution. After developing complete programs on requested topics, many inservice educators are frustrated to find attendance at the meetings very small and limited. If hospital and nursing administration do not value nursing inservice as important to the professional growth of the registered nurse, this attitude will be conveyed to nursing personnel. The nursing staff will internalize the apathy and complacency of administration and establish learning goals accordingly.

The inservice educator has a very difficult task in providing the types and variety of programs necessary for staff development. Programs should be developed according to the expressed needs of the nursing staff, as well as cover those topics deemed vital to the functioning of the agency. The inservice educator must be innovative and provide programs that are interesting, stimulating, and motivating. This, too, can only be accomplished if the educator has a philosophy that incorporates creativity as a major component.

One of the primary responsibilities of the inservice coordinator is that of developing and implementing orientation programs for new graduates. A stock orientation program is easier for the inservice to administer but will rarely meet all the needs of the individuals involved in the program. The program must be flexible enough for each graduate to increase skills in those areas he or she identifies as needing development. The inservice educator must rise to the challenge of adapting the orientation program to meet each individual's unique educational needs.

Most traditional orientation programs include a set of group activities in which the new graduate must participate. This includes administering medications for a selected number of clients, beginning with a small number and increasing to a larger group when appropriate. Another planned experience places the "technical" graduate by the bedside so that care can actually be practiced, while the educator evaluates the strengths and weaknesses of the learner's technical skills.

After a short period with the client, the graduate is usually rotated to numerous agency departments for an introduction to the essentials of each. A large amount of information is disseminated in a relatively short period of time. Finally, most orientation programs include a brief exposure to management techniques. This is accomplished in most instances by having the new graduate follow around after the head nurse and/or team leader in an effort to learn the function of various supervisory personnel.

This type of orientation does not meet the needs of the individual graduate and does not afford the opportunity for self-understanding, self-direction, self-planning and self-evaluation—characteristics essential for the professional nurse who wishes to practice nursing with excellence.

The creative orientation program provides an opportunity for value clarification for the new graduate. By requiring new graduates to list priorities for the new learning and employment experience, the inservice educator can formulate individualized educational plans. For example, a graduate may indicate the need to improve a certain technical skill instead of visiting various agency departments as originally planned in the orientation program. This type of stock orientation program would also not be appropriate for individuals who had prior work experience in the agency. Thus, each experience should be evaluated for its worth to the individual graduate, not its intended worth as determined by the institution. Conferences should be held between the head nurse or preceptor and the new graduate in order to establish open dialogue and determine the graduate's priorities and learning needs so the inservice educator can provide pertinent learning opportunities in the future.

New graduates should be able to choose their assignments for the day. The graduate must be held accountable for both client selection and nursing practice. This opportunity for freedom of choice would support the graduate in assuming responsibility for furthering his or her learning experience in order to provide high-quality nursing care to the consumer. The inservice educator and the head nurse or preceptor can facilitate the education of the new graduate during orientation and should be encouraged to maximize the learner's potential at every opportunity.

CREATIVE CLINICAL STRATEGIES

The nurse educator must select those teaching strategies that provide the student with the best learning opportunities. Creative teaching strategies should be based on the following principles:

The learner as a responsible thinking being. Teaching strategies should be consistent with the philosophy of the nursing program that views the learner as a sensing, thinking unity who is responsible and goal directed. These concepts should then be reflected in curriculum objectives, conceptual framework, level objectives, and course content. An example of this approach is shown in Exhibit 5–2.

The teaching strategies relevant to the concepts of self-direction, inquiry or questioning, and freedom of choice must be utilized in all levels of instruction. In the clinical setting the teacher would have to encourage goal setting by the student and independent decision making when appropriate. Learning experiences through inquiry, discovery, and exploration must be the goal of all instruction.

Specific clinical objectives. Teaching strategies should be related to the objectives of the specific clinical focus. There should be a direct correlation between the theoretical content of the course and the clinical objectives for the week in which the material is being taught. Teaching strategies should be selected so as to reinforce the course content while meeting the clinical objectives for each clinical experience (see Exhibit 5–3).

Teaching strategies related to the clinical focuses listed in Exhibit 5–3 must provide the student with active learning experiences in assessing the client with nutritional deficiencies or special needs. This clinical setting provides a variety of learning experiences that can be introduced to the student. Diet histories can be obtained from clients in various age groups and with many different health concerns. Comparisons can be made and students can prepare for nutritional teaching for each client.

Individual student goals. Teaching strategies should meet the needs of the learner according to established teacher-learner education goals. The student's education behavior is greatly influenced not only by past, present, and expected future experiences, but also by motivation, desire, and effort to learn. The student's educational goals will vary greatly according to each of these factors. Exhibit 5–4 represents three students' individual goals in a unit on mobility.

The teacher must be sufficiently flexible in choosing strategies for various students to meet their established educational goals for a day's experience. The inservice educator must also collaborate with new graduates to establish their individual learning needs. A group of graduates going through the same orientation program will have many different goals. They must be told of the experiences available and helped to decide which would best meet the needs they have identified.

Creative teaching. Teaching methods should be selected according to the teacher's ability to use them effectively. Traditional teaching methods are often the only strategies that the teacher utilizes. Besides the obvious reasons for this— comfort, stability, and security—the teacher often can see no alternatives in the

Exhibit 5–2 Curriculum Objectives

Upon completion of the nursing program the graduate

Demonstrates self-direction.
Assumes responsibility for own behavior.
Uses inquiry in establishing strategies for nursing care.

Conceptual Framework:

Concept	Subconcept	Theoretical Framework
Human beings	Unidirectionally	M. Rogers [6]
	Sentience	M. Rogers [7]
	Freedom of choice	C.R. Rogers [8]
Nursing	Inquiry	F. Abdellah [9]

Level Objectives:

First Level

After completing the first level of the nursing program, the student

a. Demonstrates self-direction.
b. Develops principles of inquiry.
c. Applies principles of inquiry.
d. Assumes responsibility for own behavior.

Second Level

After completing the second level of the nursing program, the student

a. Demonstrates self-direction.
b. Uses inquiry in applying concepts of nursing.
c. Assumes responsibility for own behavior.

Third Level

After completing the third level of the nursing program, the student

a. Demonstrates self-direction.
b. Uses inquiry in establishing strategies for nursing care.
c. Assumes responsibility for own behavior.

Course Content:

Concept of person
  a. Definition
  b. Awareness of self
    1. Thinking, sensing, questioning
    2. Self-direction
    3. Freedom of choice
    4. Body image or self-concept

Exhibit 5–3 Course Content

Class Content	*Nutritional Needs*
Nursing Assessment	The student will
1. Age and sex	1. Describe how age and sex affect nutritional needs.
2. Body frame and weight	2. Determine how body frame and weight affect nutritional needs.
3. Diet history	3. Explain the importance of a diet history in nursing assessment.
4. Oral cavity	4. Relate how alterations of the oral cavity affect human resources.
5. Diagnostic studies	5. Describe the diagnostic study related to nutritional needs.

Clinical Focus
1. Assess the nutritional needs of the client.
2. Obtain a diet history.
3. Review the diagnostic test of the client.
4. Compare the diagnostic results with the clinical picture of the client's health problem.
5. Make a nursing diagnosis based on the nursing assessment.

Exhibit 5–4 Teaching Strategies To Meet Three Students' Goals

Student 1
Goal: To develop proficiency in nursing techniques related to mobility.
Strategy: The student would demonstrate competencies in such activities as transfer methods, crutch walking, range of motion exercises, and positioning.

Student 2
Goal: To provide support to the client exhibiting emotional stress related to immobility.
Strategy: The student would demonstrate good communication skills, and provide perceptual stimulation.

Student 3
Goal: To demonstrate preventative and rehabilitative nursing care related to immobility.
Strategy: The student would develop a plan of care and write nursing orders related to potential complications of the immobile client.

educational setting. To shout "Be creative. Provide active learning experiences" without providing appropriate inservice education in this area is futile.

A teacher who is expected to teach creatively but who has never used inquiry as a strategy of teaching should, in most cases, not choose this method of teaching. To use the method effectively, one must develop skill in its use and application. This responsibility for educating teachers in the use of creative and active learning strategies falls within the realm of faculty and nursing inservice committees. It is therefore imperative that if teachers are expected to use certain teaching strategies they must first learn to use them effectively.

Creative and effective learning tools. The main purpose of any teaching strategy is to institute a change in the behavior of the student. If this is not accomplished then the teaching strategy, no matter how creative, is ineffectual. It is important for the clinical teacher to remember this when trying to promote creativity in the student. Just as there is rarely one answer to any given question, there is rarely only one teaching strategy for any given learning situation. The selection of each strategy must be based on all of the foregoing criteria and every attempt should be made by the teacher to apply the strategies creatively. A variety of teaching methods tends to stimulate learning in the student, although this is not necessary for effective behavioral change to take place. On the other hand, creative teaching techniques, if not presented appropriately, will have the opposite effect on the student. The clinical teacher must carefully decide how to approach each learning experience, striving always to promote maximum learning.

Clinical Conferences

It is impossible to discuss teaching strategies without including the value of pre- and post-conferences as creative teaching tools. Pre- and post-conferences are group learning experiences that occur as an integral part of the day's clinical experience. They each have definite purposes and essential components that can be utilized creatively by the instructor to provide exceptional learning experiences. Both the instructor and students must take particular responsibility to ensure that each conference provides a basis for further growth toward accomplishment of curriculum objectives.

The teacher has a responsibility to the students to be the group leader, facilitator, and energizer. The teacher directs the students' activities during the conference by (1) identifying the major areas of content and discussion, (2) relating material discussed to the clinical focus and theoretical content of the course, (3) identifying new learning needs of the students, and (4) providing opportunities for inquiry concerning unanswered questions and unresolved issues.

Students should be taught to defend their choices of care on the basis of fact rather than inferences. They should be encouraged to express their feelings about care of their clients and to clarify the points of view they express. As part of the process of inquiry, the teacher must explore with the students alternatives in nursing interventions relating to the nursing diagnosis. Decision making and freedom of choice should be consistently interwoven into every clinical conference.

As the clinical instructor, the nursing teacher must deal with problems related to group process in clinical conferences. Common problems in group interactions are conflict, apathy, and nonparticipation. Conflicts within a group are often the result of hard task assignments that the students feel are impossible for them to complete. Their own interests may conflict with those of the group, or their interests may be directed toward their own goals rather than those of the group. Apathy within a group is often a problem that the nurse educator must deal with in clinical conferences. It may occur because of a lack of interest of one or more of the group's members or a great interest in other activities or thoughts. This problem must be identified and acknowledged by the leader before any change in student behavior can occur. The group can then solve the problem of apathy by free expression of feelings and concerns. Nonparticipation may be a concern to the instructor when several individuals within the group fail to become actively involved in the group discussion. Group members should be encouraged to contribute to the group process, and every attempt should be made by the instructors to promote equal participation by all the students.

Pre-conference

The pre-conference is a combination group discussion and planning session immediately preceding an assigned clinical learning experience lasting from 30 to 60 minutes. The purposes of the pre-conference are to (1) provide direction for learning for the day utilizing the clinical focus, (2) lay the groundwork for analysis in post-conference of the day's experiences, (3) identify the scope and limitations of the nurses' role in relation to the day's clinical assignment, and (4) provide additional opportunity to identify with the nursing process. The instructor must be prepared to discuss with the students any questions they may pose related to assisting their clients with health care. Students must come to the conference prepared to discuss how their educational goals relate to their client assignments. They have an idea what significance the learning experience will have for them and what intellectual processes will be needed to accomplish their clinical objectives. They should also have reviewed the theoretical content applicable to the clinical focus and their assigned clients. As a result of this expectation, the teacher must also be knowledgeable about the students' individual educational goals and clinical objectives. This may well take hours of preparation on the part of both teacher and student.

The pre-conference is the time when the students relate their previously made assessments and nursing diagnoses to the day's clinical focus. Discussion should include the assessment data collected and questions related to the newly formulated nursing care plan. Teacher and student can collaborate on the nursing orders they prescribe for the clients and discuss alternative methods of care. The entire pre-conference should be a time of sharing and comparing ideas, nursing techniques, and creative plans for nursing care.

Some faculty prefer to forego the group pre-conference for individual pre-conferences. With this method all the students can begin to care for their clients while the educator meets with each student individually. The group sharing and comparing would take place at the post-conference. Individual pre-conferencing can be a beneficial alternative to regular pre-conferences because (1) it provides the educator with an opportunity to direct individual students in private, (2) students have more time to spend with their clients without sacrificing a planning session, and (3) the educator can privately evaluate the quality of the students' preparation.

It is recommended that this type of pre-conference be used with discretion and that pre-conferences be the common practice. A mixture of each type of conferencing provides the students with optimum learning experiences.

The new graduate should also be afforded a time to discuss the day's goals with his or her preceptor. The activities planned can be reviewed and questions asked prior to care. The preceptor can then estimate how much supervision will be required. Helping the learner establish priorities may lessen the feeling ''I wish I had had more time to . . .'' at the end of the day.

Post-conference

The post-conference immediately follows an assigned clinical learning experience and is a time for students to discuss and evaluate client care. Students and teacher also analyze the clinical learning experience, with the teacher clarifying the relationship between theory and practice while focusing on the themes of the conceptual framework. This conference also reinforces previous learning and provides an opportunity for the student to grow in the nursing process. Post-conferences should be a mandatory component of clinical instruction and not left to the discretion of an instructor.

Post-conferences can be organized with varying topics such as:

- those selected prior to the semester by the faculty team, e.g., corticosteroid therapy, conflict management
- those dictated by the objectives of the weekly clinical focus

- situations that arise unexpectedly on the clinical setting that warrant discussion

It is the responsibility of the student to discuss with peers the effectiveness of the day's plan of care, comparing the day's actual nursing care experiences with the planned experiences. Possible revisions of the nursing care plan can be suggested that would better assist the client in maintaining a desired level of well-being. The student should also share with the other students any theoretical content that applies to the day's activities. During post-conference the students discuss client nursing diagnosis and the related nursing orders. Validation of the previously made assessment, nursing diagnoses, and nursing orders is a very important part of this conference period.

The post-conference between new graduate and preceptor provides a private time for sharing. Even if a unit is extremely busy, ten minutes can always be found for this conference in which the learner can share triumphs and tribulations with a responsive listener. The preceptor can help the learner to identify factors that may have contributed to dissatisfaction and to differentiate the ones that could have been controlled from those that could not. It is at this time that specific accomplishments can be highlighted. The post-conference can be a great comfort to the new graduate, who often feels overwhelmed by the end of a shift.

Since pre- and post-conferences in themselves can be very structured and inflexible, the instructor must strive to make the interaction as stimulating and innovative as possible. Creative instruction not only is beneficial to the student for maintaining interest during the conference, but also emphasizes creativity as being vital to nursing education as well as nursing service. Creative teaching strategies must be utilized in addition to the basic group discussion for creative learning to occur.

Nursing Rounds

One teaching strategy that provides the student with the opportunity to transfer and apply the knowledge received in the classroom and college laboratory to the clinical setting is nursing rounds. The major difference between this method and other forms of instruction is the presence of the client, or third party, in the teaching-learning situation. In nursing rounds the health care consumer is the focus of clinical instruction. The strategy is based upon the premise that since the action related to health care is at the bedside, so should the learning be. The nurse educator and the nursing students visit the clients on a unit to discuss their problems and nursing care. There the instructor and students have the opportunity to exchange ideas with each client regarding how to improve client care and well-being.

This method of instruction certainly provides students with the opportunity to view a large variety of clients, listen to their concerns, and see their problems and equipment. A great many nurse educators support this teaching method as an excellent means for bedside education and the development of a sharing relationship between client and student. Since students have the responsibility for leading the rounds for their respective assigned clients, they must be well prepared and knowledgeable about nursing information and about the clients. Their individual approaches to this learning experience can be as creative and effective as the imagination permits. Nursing rounds can promote creativity in the student as well as providing an excellent learning experience.

Although the concept of nursing rounds seems very educationally sound and creative, it has one defect that requires us to examine it critically. If the conceptual framework of the nursing program is based on the unity of the individual client and is directed toward clients' rights and privileges as human beings, then this teaching strategy can be said to violate that philosophy. Hospitalization for the sick or injured person, no matter how self-assured, is at best a frightening, dependent, and belittling experience. Clients must rely upon others to fulfill their needs and wants. Fear of retaliation from the nursing and medical staff as well as lack of energy often force clients to accept tests and treatments they do not want. In the submissive role of client, hospitalized people resort to going along with the desires of the nursing staff, nurse educators, doctors, and other health professionals. Nursing rounds may be just another infringement upon human rights, since clients are not sure what will happen if they refuse to allow the "group" or students to congregate around their beds for auditory and visual observations. Obtaining permission from clients prior to the experience verifies only that the clients know the students are making rounds, not that they truly wish to give permission. Unless a client has a very strong will and is more verbal than most, he or she will submit to this experience regardless of true feelings.

Many schools recognize the AHA Patient's Bill of Rights and actively incorporate it into the clinical experience of the students. This prevents the students from infringing upon the clients' rights and privileges for the sake of education. Such a policy in the nursing program might be written as follows:

Human Rights Statement

No student other than the assigned student for that client, except when additional assistance is needed, will be allowed to observe a client, procedure, or equipment. This is consistent with the American Hospital Association's Patient's Bill of Rights, 1973.

A decision concerning the use of nursing rounds as a teaching strategy must be made individually by the nurse educator as well as by the entire nursing faculty. Its use as an effective teaching strategy must be weighed with the importance of clients' rights during hospitalization. Perhaps when faculty permit or encourage more than one student to observe a client or procedure, the principle that is taught is that "it is sometimes legitimate to infringe upon or violate the privacy of a client." Certainly, faculty would agree with the danger of this principle and should carefully examine strategies in practice that in fact do violate the human rights of clients.

Family Care

Most philosophies of schools of nursing include the care of the family as well as that of the client. However, in reality, most programs place students in acute care settings during the 7 to 3 shift on selected days Monday through Friday. These experiences occur when the agencies have no visiting hours for families or when families are working and cannot visit. Thus students are prevented from making any meaningful contact with clients' families.

Interactions with families are very valuable learning experiences and students should have opportunities to work with the total family unit. Families are excellent sources for assessment data for health histories of the client as well as for the family. Family contact also enables the student to provide health education in identified areas of need.

It is not always possible or desirable for nurse educators to arrange learning experiences for students in agencies on evenings or weekends when families are present. Learning experiences should be sought that would provide opportunities for students to interact with families as well as clients. Clinical settings where this can occur include:

- Intensive care waiting rooms
- Cardiac care waiting rooms
- Surgical waiting rooms
- Obstetrical waiting rooms
- Emergency waiting rooms

Communication skills can be used to provide comfort and support to the families in crisis. Exhibit 5–5 is an example of a focus sheet for this type of experience.

Other areas where students could interact with families and clients include:

- Outpatient clinics
- Specialized clinics (Orthopedic, Antepartal, Postpartal, Diabetic, etc.)
- Well baby clinics

Exhibit 5–5 Family Care—Crisis

FOCUS: Situational Crisis

1. Assess the family's coping abilities.
2. Identify the family's support system.
3. Identify nursing diagnoses related to the family situation.
4. Relate the crisis situation to the grieving process.
5. Identify areas of need for health education and information.

- Family planning clinics
- Family clinics
- Homes of friends and/or relatives
- Community agencies (Visiting Nurses, Public Health, senior citizen groups, etc.)

The student can assess the interactions between the client and family members as well as provide health education to the group. Exhibit 5–6 is an example of a focus sheet for this type of learning experience.

Assessment

Assessment is a skill that is often difficult to learn. One reason for this may be the large amount of extraneous information available as data sources. To compensate for misuse of these data, the educator can assign students to clients without allowing them to use the medical records for data collection. This strategy refines the assessment skills of the student since all data gathered have to come from subjective and/or objective observations. This can be done with or without

---

Exhibit 5–6 Family Care—Well-Being

FOCUS: Developmental Situation

1. Assess the family for developmental levels.
2. Identify family structure (i.e., nuclear, extended, homosexual, etc.).
3. Assess family functions (include roles and communication patterns).
4. Identify areas of need for health education.
5. Select one individual and complete a developmental assessment.

---

informing the student of the client's medical diagnosis. (Of course, the student should be informed of the essential data needed to provide safe care such as diet, activity level, oxygen, etc.). The advantage of this strategy is that all information gathered will not be biased by opinions, inferences, and irrelevant data documented by other nursing and medical personnel. This activity usually results in accurate observations for the assessment and information that reveals the clients' views of their illness, treatments, prognoses, etc. It also promotes the importance of the client's input into the nursing process.

Another aspect of the same strategy is for the educator to assign one student to a client for a total health history with no input from the medical records. Another student is assigned to the same client but has no contact with the client and/or family. The first student will obtain all the data from the client and family and the second student can use only the records and other health care personnel for information. The students complete their assigned tasks and bring the information to post-conference. At this time comparisons are made between the data collected from the client and that derived from the records and staff members. Students who are involved in this experience will benefit from the results of these two methods of data collection.

This activity assists students in identifying sources of information pertinent to the assessment process and those that provide inaccurate or irrelevant data. The students will gather data from the feelings and perceptions of the client and be able to compare this information with that documented in or absent from the medical records. In many instances, nurses treat the client according to what the records indicate is wrong and not what the client perceives as being the problem. It is recommended that these assignments be made for all students on the unit. These experiences will reinforce the fact that clients are truly experts on their own well-being.

Nursing Care Patterns

A very difficult part of the student's education is the transition from the "total client care" philosophy to the realities of the work world. In order to reinforce the importance of continuity of care, individualized care, and quality care, the following teaching strategies can be used. The students are assigned to care for a number of clients according to the functional method of providing care. That is, one or two students bathe the clients, one or two students make the beds, one or two students pass medications, etc. This can be done for only one day, although several days of this experience will provide a more accurate example of the type of nursing care offered with this staffing pattern. Following this experience, the group of students are then assigned to care for the clients as a team. Caution must be taken to prevent the team nursing method from developing into functional nursing care.

Last, the students are assigned to clients using primary or modular nursing methods of staffing. The students should keep a nursing log of all their experiences and feelings about the care they provided. It would be beneficial for the students also to record the reactions of the client to the care and their own evaluations of the quality of the care given in each care pattern. At the end of the experience, the information from the students is compared and an evaluation of the methods is made.

Another method of enlightening students as to the components of quality nursing care is for the educator to assign one client to each student in one-half the group and two or more clients to the other half of students. The students from each group compare the quality of care given to the clients during the experience. In post-conference they should share what they did for their client or clients, what care could or could not be given as a result of time constraints, and what level of care was administered.

This experience demonstrates to students that caring for more than one or two clients results in less client contact and, therefore, less client care. It assists students in realizing that priorities have to be established when time constraints do not allow for all aspects of nursing care to be given. Selecting specific nursing interventions for care is a difficult task for students who usually have time to do almost everything for the client. This experience promotes growth in decision making and establishing priorities of care.

Other Strategies

Nursing faculty who desire to be creative in their clinical instruction can assist each other by brainstorming to develop innovative learning experiences for their students. The following are selected strategies that can be used by the creative instructor.

- Orient students to a unit through a treasure hunt.
- Assign students to teach a client or clients about a health subject. Do not assign any aspect of physical care.
- Assign two students to make assignments for a number of other students in the group. They must do this task according to the clinical focus and the educational needs of the learner.
- Direct the students to make their own assignments according to their own learning needs.
- Direct the students to randomly select a client after visiting with several individuals.
- Develop creative learning activities on specific topics. Exhibit 5–7 illustrates a creative learning activity related to pain.

Exhibit 5–7 Creative Learning Activity Related to Pain

FOCUS: Learning Activities Related to Pain

1. Interview a client who has had pain.
2. Discuss students' perceptions of how it feels to do a painful procedure on a client.
3. Debate the use of placebos.
4. Role play a personal experience with pain.
5. Observe two clients experiencing pain of the same type (i.e., insertion of an IV). Compare the clients' reactions.
6. Interview practicing registered nurses regarding their attitudes about pain and pain relief.
7. Interview clients as to their methods of coping with pain.   •

SUMMARY

Clinical instruction in nursing, a specialized method of teaching, can occur in any health care system of society. The most frequent place for clinical instruction is in the hospital setting, although more and more nursing programs are utilizing community facilities effectively. The change from teaching nursing exclusively in acute care settings has occurred as a result of the changing patterns of society. Although most clinical teaching is still located in the hospital, 90 percent of individuals who need or desire health care are neither hospitalized nor acutely ill. The age of anxiety and affluence has directed health care toward the emotional and physical well-being of the individual outside of the hospital climate and into the community. These trends in nursing education make it imperative that more attention be paid to the clinical teacher and strategies for effective and creative clinical instruction.

SUGGESTED READINGS

Clark, Carolyn Chambers. "Simulation Gaming: A New Teaching Strategy in Nursing Education." *Nurse Educator* (November/December 1976):4–9.

Cooper, Signe, S. "Methods of Teaching—Revisited." *Journal of Continuing Education in Nursing* 9 (July/August 1978):24–25.

———. "Methods of Teaching—Revisited; Brainstorming." *Journal of Continuing Education in Nursing* 9 (November/December 1978):16–18.

———. "Methods of Teaching—Revisited; Games and Simulation." *Journal of Continuing Education in Nursing* 10 (September/October 1979):14, 47–48.

———. "Methods of Teaching—Revisited; Informal Discussion." *Journal of Continuing Education in Nursing* 9 (September/October 1978):14–16.

———. "Methods of Teaching—Revisited; Nursing Care Conference." *Journal of Continuing Education in Nursing* 10 (January/February 1979):28–30.

deTournay, Rheba. *Strategies for Teaching Nursing*. New York: John Wiley, 1971.

Hahn, Robert O. *Creative Teachers: Who Wants Them?* New York: John Wiley, 1973.

Holm, Karyn, et al. "A Teaching-Learning Experience: Nursing Rounds." *Journal of Nursing Education* 17 (April 1978):33–36.

Holt, John. *Freedom and Beyond*. New York: E.P. Dutton, 1972.

Kagan, Jerome (ed.). *Creativity and Learning*. Boston: Houghton Mifflin, 1967.

Lundsteen, Sara W. "Questioning To Develop Creative Problem Solving." *Elementary English* 51 (May 1974):645–650.

Lytton, Hugh. *Creativity and Education*. New York: Schocken Books, 1972.

Mereness, Dorothy. "Freedom and Responsibility for Nursing Students." *American Journal of Nursing* 67 (January 1967):69–71.

Michael, William B. (ed.). *Teaching for Creative Endeavor: Bold New Venture*. Bloomington, Ind.: Indiana University Press, 1968.

Miel, Alice (ed.). *Creativity in Teaching*. Belmont, Calif.: Wadsworth, 1961.

O'Shea, Helen Spustek, and Margaret Kidd Parsons. "Clinical Instruction; Effective and Ineffective Teaching Behavior." *Nursing Outlook* 27 (June 1979):411–415.

Schweer, Jean E., and Kristine M. Gebbie. *Creative Teaching in Clinical Nursing*. St. Louis: C.V. Mosby, 1976.

Smith, Dorothy W. *Perspectives on Clinical Teaching*. New York: Springer, 1968.

Steele, Shirley, and Frank L. Maraviglia. *Creativity in Nursing*. Thorofare, N.J.: Charles B. Slack, 1981.

Taylor, Sandra, Mary S. Brodish, and Hazel N. Brown. "Creative Learning Experience for Student Nurses." *Journal of Nursing Education* 18, no. 4 (April 1979):16–18.

Thomas, Barbara. "Promoting Creativity in Nursing Education." *Nursing Research* 28, no. 2 (March-April 1979):115–119.

Wold, Zane Robinson, and Rose Woytowich O'Driscoll. "How Useful Is the Preclinical Conference?" *Nursing Outlook* 27 (July 1979):455–457.

Chapter 6

Preparation for Clinical Instruction

Nursing is learned by a process of interaction with the instructor, especially in the clinical experience. Classroom objectives are formulated in order to address specific concepts and content within the curriculum. The learning objectives for an agency orientation program should likewise be derived from the philosophy of the institution and selected according to what the agency deems necessary for the successful practice of nursing.

Preparation for classroom teaching is lengthy—usually a minimum of three hours of preparation to every hour of classroom instruction. With thorough preparation the educator can select material that will best promote understanding of the topics to be covered. The creative classroom teacher can promote the students' interest in learning by providing opportunities for individual choice and exploration.

Unfortunately, the nurse educator often does not realize that clinical teaching, too, requires thorough preparation. Many who agree that the clinical experience is very significant fail to equate the behavioral outcomes of clinical learning with the teacher's preparation or lack of it. Clinical learning must be a planned activity and contain opportunities and experiences essential for quality education.

CLINICAL OBJECTIVES

Clinical objectives reflect the expected student behavior desired at the conclusion of the clinical course. They evolve directly from the classroom objectives and content. Exhibit 6–1 illustrates the evolution of clinical objectives and focus objectives from the curriculum.

Clinical objectives serve to:

- define the desired learning outcomes (cognitive, affective, psychomotor skills)

Exhibit 6–1 Evolution of Clinical Objectives

UNIT OBJECTIVES

1. Assess the needs of the client and family related to structural mobility.
2. Establish a plan of care with the client and family related to the nursing diagnoses of mobility structure needs.
3. Assist the client and family with mobility structure needs.
4. Evaluate a plan of care related to mobility structure needs.

Class Content:

1. Nursing Assessment
   - Motor Strength
   - Range of Motion
   - Activities of Daily Living
   - Diagnostic Studies
2. Nursing Diagnoses
   - Impaired Physical Mobility
3. Planning
   - Body Image
   - Capacity To Function
4. Nursing Implementation
   - Nursing Intervention
   - Medication
   - Rehabilitation
5. Medical Diagnoses Related to Nursing Diagnoses
   - Definition
   - Clinical Characteristics
   - Medical Intervention
   - Surgical Procedures

Clinical Focus Objectives

General Objectives:

1. Assess the mobility structure needs of the client.
2. Review diagnostic results with the client.
3. Develop a plan of care related to mobility structure needs.
4. Describe the nursing interventions related to mobility structure needs.
5. Evaluate a plan of care related to mobility structure needs.

Specific Objectives:

1. Assess the client for problems in mobility.
2. Identify the client's deviation in mobility.
3. Discuss with the client the hazards of mobility.
4. Describe those nursing interventions used to prevent the hazards of mobility.
5. Establish health goals related to mobility.
6. Assist the client with achievement of established health goals.
7. Evaluate the success of achievement of health goals with the client.

- direct the selection of clinical settings
- guide the selection of student assignments
- organize teaching-learning activities
- measure students' level of performance

Clinical Focus Guidelines

Clinical focus guidelines are explicit learning objectives tailored to direct the learner to daily learning activities in the clinical setting. Focus objectives are derived directly from the broad course clinical objectives. Focus objectives ensure that each learner will be provided with the opportunity to learn the content that has been determined as primary by the faculty. Exhibit 6–2 outlines the purpose and format of focus objectives.

The format consists of general and specific objectives. The general objectives encompass the broad overall goals for the experience. The guideline then outlines specific objectives and activities to direct the learner.

The number of clinical focus guidelines for a particular clinical course will be dependent upon the total number of clinical sessions (hours, days). If a clinical course has 16 clinical days, 12 clinical focus guidelines could be formulated. This would leave 4 days without specific guidelines. Clinical days without specific focus guidelines would be utilized to:

- allow the learner to complete a previous focus guideline that was missed because of absence or an unavailable client assignment.
- provide the instructor with opportunities to utilize clinical time for a specific goal or to discuss a specific client situation.

The learner would receive all the clinical focus guidelines at the beginning of the clinical period. Each learner would know which guideline would be utilized each day.

The learner keeps the guideline and records appropriate data. During the post-conference session, each student will contribute data to the overall discussion of the focus topic. The instructor can review the completed form at indicated times.

Since the learner is often rotated into a particular setting or experience, a different focus guideline would direct the learner in that experience while the other learners would be focusing on another guideline. For example:

Learner 1   Clinical Focus Guideline for OR Experience
Learner 2   Clinical Focus Guideline for Client Education Experience
Learners 3–10 Clinical Focus Guidelines for Neurosensory Assessment

Learners 1 and 2 would be required to complete the focus guidelines on neuro-sensory assessment on another day.

Focus objectives are especially useful in directing the learner during experiences when the instructor is not present, as in peri-operative or day care center assignments.

Exhibit 6–2 Clinical Focus Objectives Format

Purpose:

- To direct the learner toward a specific goal with explicit learning objectives.
- To provide for planned learning opportunities rather than relying on incidental learning.
- To control the changing variables on the clinical unit that can interfere with learning.
- To assist the educator with making assignments.

Format:

General Objectives (Examples)

- Observe the physical setup of the nursing unit
- Assess the nutritional status of the individual
- Identify the client's alterations related to respiratory function

Specific Objectives (Examples)

- Observe the nursing unit (general, OR, DR, ER, etc.) or a community agency
  physical setup
  safety precautions
  equipment (routine, emergency)
  procedures
  policies
- Assess for selected data

comfort	dysfunctions
skin	cardiac
nutrition	circulatory
safety	respiratory
mobility	renal
elimination	neurosensory
emotional status	musculoskeletal
coping patterns	gastrointestinal
relationship patterns	

- Perform a specific intervention
  A.M. care
  dressing change
  pre/post operative care
  communication technique
  newborn care
  physical assessment
    skin
    vital signs
- Prepare for selected experiences (medications, team leader, OR, community agency)
  assign readings
  prior visit
- Evaluate
  effectiveness of the care
  response of the client

The focus objectives clearly outline the goals and responsibilities of the learner and reduce instances where the learner "missed" the learning. Appendix 6–A illustrates an example of a clinical focus guideline for an observational experience.

Clinical Focus Guidelines for Staff Nurses

Clinical focus guidelines can be utilized to orient new staff to an agency. Knowledge and experience of the "needed to know" nature are identified by the nursing education department. Focus guidelines are created and the new employee is presented with the guidelines on day one. The learner then assumes the responsibility to acquire the experience and also to submit the completed guideline. If additional assistance is needed, the focus guidelines can direct the educator to the problem areas. Exhibit 6–3 illustrates examples of topics for clinical focus guidelines for professional orientation.

The learner can be requested to submit completed guidelines to the instructor or to compile them in a notebook that the instructor has ready access to. If a program does not utilize focus sheets as part of the clinical experience, it would be prudent for the instructors to develop them for use by their assigned students. The instructor can initially develop three or four guidelines and then proceed to develop additional guidelines as time permits. Although a time-consuming task, it should prove worth the effort because of the resulting ease in making assignments and because of the improved quality of learning. No longer will necessary learning be left to chance.

The Appendixes contain sample focus objective guidelines (Appendix 6–A), an example for a four-week experience on a mental health unit (Appendix 6–B), and an example of leveling one topic from simple to complex in four courses (Appendix 6–C).

Exhibit 6–3 Examples of Clinical Focus Guidelines for Professional
Orientation

- Observation of unit (physical setup, personnel, traffic pattern)
- Admission to unit
- Nursing physical assessment (see Chapter 7 for topical outline)
- Initiation of a care plan
- Pre/post operative care
- Discharge from unit
- Community referrals
- Equipment use
- Documentation

SELECTION OF UNIT OR AGENCY FOR CLINICAL TEACHING

The establishment of clinical objectives and focus guidelines leads to the selection of the unit or agency. Clinical settings are selected where students will have the clinical experiences that will provide them with the opportunity to attain the desired learning.

Presently, schools of nursing utilize a variety of clinical settings to prepare the student for the expanded roles of professional nursing. Faculty need to proceed cautiously in the selection of clinical sites. Since the majority of professional nurses practice in acute care settings, how much clinical experience in other settings (community health centers, schools, etc.) is appropriate without sacrificing the learning of critical practice skills? Exhibit 6–4 represents the result of a study of 90 BSN schools to determine the type of clinical sites being used.

The following questions may assist faculty with the selection of a clinical facility or in evaluating the appropriateness of a present clinical site:

- Does the client population provide the variety of experiences necessary to attain clinical focus objectives?
- What is the quality of care delivered at the setting?
- Are there sufficient numbers of clients to accommodate the clinical group?

Exhibit 6–4 Types of Clinical Sites in Order of Percentage of Use in BSN Programs

Secondary Care Settings
Homes
Health Departments
Tertiary Care Settings
Schools
Community Mental Health Agencies
Day Care Centers
Home Health Agencies
Rehabilitation Centers
Physician Offices
Industries
Community Action Programs
Health Maintenance Organizations
Jails
Summer Camps

Source: B.A. Graham and C.J. Gleit, "Clinical Sites Used in Baccalaureate Programs," *Nursing Outlook* 29 (May 1981): 291–294.

- What is the response of personnel to students?
- What is the philosophy of the agency concerning students, faculty, and nontraditional learning experiences?
- How have past students evaluated the facility?
- Will students have access to and use of records (Kardex, charts, care plans)? patient care conferences? consultations (staff, physicians, social service, nutritionists, etc.)?
- Will students be permitted to provide all aspects of nursing care (medications, treatments, assessments)?
- Is the facility available for use during the designated period (days, hours)?
- How accessible is the clinical facility (travel, safety)?
- How utilized is the agency by other student groups?
- What is the major reason for selecting the facility or a nontraditional experience (convenience, faculty preference, variety of experiences, placement of "extra" students, established contractual agreements)?

SELECTION OF UNIT FOR EMPLOYEE ORIENTATION

Orientation programs within hospitals or other health care agencies often use units that are not conducive to learning and educational objectives. Which unit is selected for orientation of new graduates or new employees often depends upon the staffing patterns of the institution and the staffing needs of that unit. Units that are short-handed are often selected for orientation of new employees. But this is unfortunate because in most cases a unit with staffing deficiencies not only would *not* benefit from the added stress of orienting a new employee but also might detract from the experience for the new nurse.

Units with high turnover rates should be examined closely before they are utilized for an orientation program. Possible reasons for rapid turnover should be investigated for diagnosis and treatment of the problem. The policy for placing new employees, especially new graduates, on a unit where their resignation is predictable, should certainly be questioned.

To avoid the use of potential problem units, a survey of attitudes and values could be conducted to find which units within an agency might support the orientation of new graduates and add to their educational experience. Criteria for selection might include client/staff ratios, attitudes about nursing and education, and an acceptance of new and progressive trends. The success of the new graduate or employee is nurtured in an environment where professional staff function as goal-directed facilitators.

One technique for enhancing orientation of new employees is the *preceptorship program*. The preceptor, an experienced staff nurse, is assigned to guide a new employee through the orientation process. The preceptor should be given classes on the principles of teaching and learning as well as methods and strategies of education. Since the professional staff nurse must be available to support and guide the new graduate, it is essential that both be scheduled to work the same shifts. A one-to-one basis is the best arrangement because of the need to develop a trusting relationship between the health professional and the new employee.

COMPLETION OF CONTRACTUAL AGREEMENTS

After selection of the unit or agency for the clinical experience, a contractual agreement must be developed between the educational institution and the health care institution. The necessity for such a contract will not be detailed here, but there obviously are legal implications for both parties. Whether a contract is needed depends upon the nature of the experience to be offered to the students. Simple observation tends not to demand any formal agreement. However, this decision should be left to the individuals accountable for such decisions within both institutions.

The responsibility for negotiating the contract rests with the administration of the educational institution. To plan for the learning experiences to be covered by the contract, representatives of the health agency and the educational institution should meet. Applicability of the contract to each party should be considered and potential problems identified and discussed. Sample contractual agreements for agencies and for preceptors are provided in Appendixes 6–D and 6–E.

ORGANIZATION OF PLANNING CONFERENCES

After the mutual expectations of the institutions have been considered and contents of the contract have been established, the nurse educator should begin to plan the clinical experience in detail. If an agency or new unit is to be utilized for the first time by the educational program, it is imperative that the nurse educator begin formal preparation at least two months prior to offering the clinical experience.

The educator should meet with the appropriate supervisor and head nurse from the agency to discuss the educational objectives of the clinical experience. The initial meeting should take place on the unit so that the educator can become familiar with the physical layout of the facility. At the same time the nurse educator can also meet the nursing personnel on the unit and see what type of client population is receiving care. This information will enable the educator to assess how much students might be expected to gain from orientation on the unit.

A date for the next meeting should be scheduled at this time, with the agency given the opportunity to choose the time and place, preferably someplace where discussion can occur privately and without interruptions. The educator should follow up the initial conference with a memorandum to the agency members summarizing the meeting's discussions and confirming the date and time of the next gathering. The educator should also include a brief agenda of the topics to be covered at the next conference. Copies of schedules, course objectives, and any other pertinent information can be forwarded with this correspondence. This would allow participants sufficient time to review the material prior to the meeting and formulate questions.

If areas of conflict are known, the educator may mention them in the memo, thus forewarning the head nurse and supervisor and anyone else involved. The manner in which conflict and change are broached can enhance or hinder the interpersonal relationships between educators and agency staff. Staff of agencies or units should not feel they must accept faculty and students without any input into the process. If feelings of powerlessness are strong in the staff members, they may inadvertently react with indifference and hostility toward the educator and students as well as the entire educational process.

The purpose of the second meeting is to share the schedule for the entire clinical experience. Agency representatives are told which days, arrival and departure times, break routines, and lunch schedules are preferred. The educator should also discuss with the head nurse and supervisor the procedures for canceling clinical sessions or reporting student illness.

Opportunity should be provided to the group to express worries or reservations they may have about the educational experience. Concern is often expressed by agency representatives about making assignments, supervising students, reporting, recording, and accounting for client care. All these issues should be resolved at this meeting and all potential problems should be brought up for discussion. Any nontraditional methods of clinical instruction to be used should be brought to the attention of the head nurse and supervisor, and any anticipated problems concerning flexibility and creativity in the educational experience should be brought to light.

The philosophy of the educational program should be reviewed, as should its application to the clinical education of the professional nursing student. The course outline and the appropriate clinical focus for each topic should be discussed in an effort to predetermine the level of clinical instruction in light of the knowledge of the nursing students. An overview of the level of student experience can provide the head nurse and supervisor with a clear picture of the abilities and skills of the students.

The inservice educator should also include such information in conferences with leaders of units to be utilized for orientation. Thus distinct guidelines for new graduate behavior can be established. New educational situations during orientation should be built upon the learner's past experiences and any known deficiencies.

Clinical goals should be discussed as they relate to the clinical focus. The educator should explain how students will be assigned to provide client care. In order to demonstrate the process of assignment, the educator can use the example of one clinical focus to show the variety of assignments that could evolve from it. If the educator utilizes a nontraditional assignment, an explanation of its methodology and use will be needed. (Nontraditional teaching strategies are addressed in Chapter 5.)

Communication channels to convey pertinent information from student to head nurse should be established. Interactions between head nurse or staff and students, between staff and instructor, and between head nurse and instructor need to be considered. Not all interactions are appropriate. Answers to such questions as "When can a student request information or assistance from a staff member?" must be explored. It is necessary to make clear that all decisions relating to student supervision must rest with the educator. Before a nurse other than the instructor supervises a student during a procedure, careful consideration must be given to its appropriateness. The responsibility for educating the nursing student should be accepted by the nurse educator. This education should be planned and implemented according to set rules, regulations, and objectives. If this process is delegated or left to other individuals, its value to the learner may be lessened. What and how a student learns is the responsibility of the nurse educator, not the nursing service.

Should an educator be unfamiliar with a certain procedure or piece of equipment, the staff can be asked to explain it to the educator and the students simultaneously. This provides the needed information while promoting better interpersonal relationships between service and education.

The educator should strive for an atmosphere of mutual respect. As a guest in the health agency and on the clinical unit, the nurse educator should make the initial approach to foster a climate conducive to learning. Open and direct communication can help limit the mistrust and fear often present during a change process.

PROVIDING AGENCY ORIENTATION FOR STUDENTS

Identifying the teacher's and the learner's respective and mutual goals is one of the first steps in the educational process. Prior to orienting the students to the unit or the health agency, the educator must hold a planning conference to discuss the objectives of the experience. Letters should be sent to all students informing them of the conference and the forthcoming orientation. A two-hour period should be designated at a convenient location for a conference. Compensatory time can be returned to the student later.

The Planning Conference

The purpose of the planning conference is to discuss the pending clinical experience. The agenda might be as follows:

1. Introduction of educator and students
2. Description of the unit(s) to be used
3. Instructor's expectations
4. Students' expectations
5. Clinical focus objectives and clinical conferences
6. Assignments
7. Evaluation
8. Written assignments

Introduction of Educator and Students

During the introduction, each person shares some personal information, e.g., family, interests, etc. Sharing of one's personal life and interests enhances mutual interest and promotes caring behaviors among the group.

Description of the Unit

The instructor will describe the size, location, and type of unit that will be the clinical setting. Topics to be considered are:

- Client population (age, types of illnesses, length of stay)
- Physical facilities
- Administration (lines of communication, philosophy, morale)
- Type of nursing care system (primary, team, functional, modular)
- Personnel (type, number)
- Documentation system (Kardex, care plan, progress notes)
- Medication administration system
- Availability of supporting departmental services (radiology, laboratory, rehabilitation, pharmacy, outpatient, etc.)

Instructor's Expectations

Instructors should reveal to the students their expectations regarding the clinical experience. To do this they may first need to ask themselves "What is important for the student to learn? What learning should be incidental? What learning should be planned? How independent should students be expected to be and how often should they consult with the instructor? When can a student function without supervision? Who is responsible for student learning?'' Answers to these and many other questions will be based on the philosophy of the nurse educator.

The educator should also be explicit about the student's responsibility to function within the rules and regulations of the program and the clinical policies. Expected attendance and the procedure for notification of illness or other reasons for nonattendance should be spelled out for the students. Student responsibility to the client, educator, health agency, and self should be discussed. Students should be given the opportunity to discuss and obtain clarification on all expectations.

Students' Expectations

The students' own expectations regarding the clinical experience should also be expressed. Establishing individual learning objectives for the clinical experience is one way of ensuring successful outcomes. A list like that in Exhibit 6–5 can be submitted to the instructor for use in individualizing the clinical experience for the student. Individual learning objectives are also a valuable tool for student self-evaluation.

Clinical Focus Objectives and Clinical Conferences

The focus objective guidelines are distributed to the learner during the planning conference. Instructions are given in the use of the guidelines and the responsibil-

---

Exhibit 6–5 Student Learning Objectives

1. During this clinical experience, I would like to focus on increasing my learning in the following:
   a.
   b.
   c.
   d.
   e.
   f.
   g.
2. The technical skills that I need to perform or refine are
   a.
   b.
   c.
   d.
   e.
   f.
   g.

Date _____   Signed _____

ity of the learner for their completion. Students are asked to keep the instructor informed of their inability to complete a guideline so that future assignments can provide the opportunity.

Pre- and post-clinical conferences will be explained regarding time, length, and purpose. The responsibilities of the learner for conferences is clearly specified.

Assignments

The specific assignment method is explained to the students. The expectations of the instructor concerning the amount and type of student preparation for clinical learning is clearly outlined by the instructor.

Evaluation

The instructor should provide students with specific criteria for evaluation of clinical performance. The instructor will review each objective on the evaluation form and provide the learner with an explanation of each objective. What constitutes a clinical failure is clearly defined. In order to function at maximum ability, the student must be aware of what to do. (See Chapter 11 for more information on clinical evaluation.)

Written Assignments

Written assignments are explained with respect to

- purpose
- format
- length
- due date

In order to assist the learner in preparation of a paper or a care plan, the instructor can place several samples of past student written assignments on reserve in the library.

Tour of Clinical Setting

After the planning conference, the students should be oriented to the clinical setting. Besides the location of the unit, they should be shown the location of common equipment, the cafeteria, the library, and the lockers. They should be introduced to the staff and be told about parking and other regulations. They will not remember every detail, but this orientation is valuable in reducing students' anxiety.

Day One

Basic nursing care is the same regardless of where it is administered. With this thought in mind, the students should be able to provide safe and competent nursing care to clients even on the first day of any clinical experience. It is nonetheless advisable to minimize stress for students by making the first day's clinical assignment lighter than usual. This would enable the student to take time to get used to the unit and its procedures. During the first few clinical experiences on any new unit, the educator must work to reduce students' stress and fear of the unknown. As students begin to concentrate on the clients rather than the physical surroundings, they will find themselves less easily intimidated by new settings.

STAFF ORIENTATION

If an orientation program is to occur on a specific unit, the inservice educator should plan a meeting with the unit's head nurse to discuss the program objectives. If several units are to be used, a joint meeting of all head nurses should be held. If a preceptor program is to be part of the orientation, the inservice educator should meet with the preceptors to establish the principles of the program. Objectives and purposes of this type of orientation program can be discussed as well as the responsibilities of all the program participants.

SELECTION OF LEARNING EXPERIENCES

Since learning is effective only if it is goal directed and meaningful to the individual student, each learner should be encouraged to take the initiative in the learning experience. Preparation for the clinical experience is essential for maximum learning. All students should receive their client assignments the day before the clinical session in order to be adequately prepared.

Some methods of assignment making are:

- instructor selects the assignments
- learner selects own assignment
- instructor primarily selects the assignments, but provides the learner with opportunities to select own assignments periodically

Instructor-Selected Assignments

Students should report to the assigned unit for one to two hours on the day before the clinical experience. After receiving their assignments from the instructor, the students should visit their respective clients to make a health assessment and obtain a nursing history. Since this is vital to the clinical experience of the student, no excuses should be accepted as to why a student could not meet with an assigned client. During this preclinical experience, the student can also review the medical records of the client, even though emphasis should be on the nursing history and the data base provided by the nurse-client interaction. The hours spent in assessing and planning on the nursing unit should be counted as clinical time. The instructor should be available to clarify questions and assist the students in directing their learning experiences.

If a class or other school obligation prevents students from participating in the preclinical activity, the educator's opportunity to enhance the learning experience through assignment making will be limited. A written assignment sheet can be distributed to the students at a specified place and time on the day before the clinical experience. If this is impossible, students should be asked to call for their assignments at their convenience on the preclinical day.

In another instructor-selected arrangement the learner receives the assignment just prior to the clinical experience. This approach is usually selected when travel to the clinical setting the day before is not feasible. With this method, the learner will not have an opportunity to prepare for the experience prior to the day. In certain settings, such as labor and delivery and outpatient departments, this is the usual arrangement. In such cases the learner should be provided with preparation time that day prior to beginning care. Reference books are available on the unit for this purpose.

Learner-Selected Assignments

The opportunity for learners to select their own assignments can be a creative and purposeful teaching-learning technique. With careful planning this method can cultivate self-directed learning. Without careful planning and supervision, many optional learning experiences may be lost.

Beginning students do not have the necessary background to select their own assignments. They often overassign themselves because they cannot identify the nursing responsibilities that the assignment entails.

The practice of routinely allowing students to select their assignments should be examined by the educator. Certain students who are mature and highly motivated will select the best learning experiences. If this student also has access to the unit prior to other students, it can be predicted that the highly desirable clients will not be available for the other students.

The educator often identifies students who should be directed to certain learning experiences. It is true that this can be done prior to assignment selection; however, the educator, because of expertise, can often identify rich learning opportunities that may not be as obvious or desirable to the learner.

Students can and should be given the opportunity to select their own assignments periodically throughout the curriculum. RN students studying for a degree in nursing are usually successful in selecting their own assignments. Whichever method of making assignments is used, the educator should strive to implement change in the educational program in order to provide learners with the opportunity to prepare for the clinical experience.

In the area of assignment selection, the educator could enlist the aid of a computer. Utilizing the course and clinical focus objectives, the educator would enter all the identified learning experiences into the computer. After each clinical experience, the students would be required to enter their weekly experience (precoded) into the computer. Prior to the next clinical setting, the instructor can take a printout, which would reflect each student's present experiences, to the clinical setting to assist in assignment making. If a modem is available, the educator can tap into the agency's computer and make assignments without traveling to the agency.

The relation between the quality of assignment making and the quality of learning is close. In formulating the assignments, the educator must consider (1) the clinical weekly focus, (2) student entry skills, (3) students' personal objectives, (4) supervision time, and (5) the complexity of the experience. For example, a student who excels in psychomotor skills should be given a chance to increase his or her abilities in health teaching. An appropriate assignment by the educator could provide the student with time to devise an individualized teaching plan for an assigned client. The assignment might include teaching a client or group of clients while excluding the physical care of the same client(s) since proficiency in this area had already been developed. Thus the student would be allowed to focus on teaching and learning without being burdened by technical procedures and irrelevant responsibilities.

Although clinical teaching has a certain element of unpredictability, the following problems are predictable if planning is insufficient in the process of assignment making:

1. Frequent "surprises" or unexpected incidences that could have been foreseen
2. Students complaining of nothing to do
3. Overburdening of students
4. Insufficient supervision due to lack of time
5. Errors resulting from insufficient supervision

Exhibit 6–6 is an example of an assignment sheet that would provide the student with the necessary data to prepare for the clinical practicum. Two copies of this sheet should be made, one for the student and one for the instructor. The student can use the copy of the assignment sheet to gather data and complete the pertinent

Exhibit 6–6 Client Assignment Sheet

STUDENT _____ DATE _____

CLIENT'S NAME _____ROOM _____ AGE _____

1. Medical diagnosis

2. Pertinent social data

3. Other coexisting health problems

4. Nursing diagnosis

5. Plan of care (medications, IUs, diet, activity level, nursing orders, treatments)

6. Additional content to review

If the institution or agency does not utilize nursing diagnoses or clients' problems, then the educator would direct the students to formulate these diagnoses the first day of clinical instruction. This provides the educator with an opportunity to direct the learner to topics and references for appropriate preparation.

---

information while the educator utilizes the original for reference related to future assignments and anecdotal notes. In order to keep the agency informed of the clinical assignments, the unit should receive a list of the students with their respective client assignments.

Students who are required to participate in a preclinical assessment practicum could complete questions 2–5 in Exhibit 6–6. Thus the instructor would provide only the information needed to direct the students according to their respective levels of experience and skills in performance. Such an assignment sheet should be used in conjunction with the weekly learning objectives. For example, students who are learning the process of deriving nursing diagnoses would not have this aspect of the data provided for them.

As the students progress through the semester or block experience, the educator should provide less and less information to them during the assignment-making process, although the time the educator spends preparing and the level of detail should never be reduced. The quality of the organization and preparation for clinical instruction can directly influence the quality of the learner's experience.

SUMMARY

Systematic preparation for clinical instruction by the educator and the learner can provide the learning experiences needed to acquire skilled clinical knowledge. Through careful faculty planning prior to clinical teaching, the learner can be directed to specific learning activities rather than relying on incidental or chance learning.

SUGGESTED READINGS

Ellis, P. "Matching Students with Clinical Experiences by Computer." *Nursing Outlook* 30 (January 1982):29–30.

Fricson, L., and B. Conahan. "A Clinical Preceptor Program: Strategy for New Graduate Orientation." *The Journal of Nursing Administration* 10 (April 1980):18–19.

Holloran, S., et al. "Bicultural Training for New Graduates." *The Journal of Nursing Administration* 10 (February 1980):17–24.

O'Shea, H., et al. "Clinical Instruction: Effective and Ineffective Teacher Behaviors." *Nursing Outlook* 27 (June 1979):411–415.

Skeath, W., et al. "Criteria To Be Used in the Selection of Clinical Areas for Basic Nursing Training." *Journal of Advanced Nursing* 4 (March 1979):169–180.

Appendix 6–A

Sample Focus Objective Guidelines

Focus Sheet for an Observational Experience

FOCUS: The Aging Process

Objectives: During an observation at a senior citizen center, the student is expected to do the following:

1. Observe the biologic changes of the aging process
2. Discuss patterns of living with a selected client
3. Identify daily activities of the selected client
4. Observe the aged during mealtime
5. Participate in specified diversional activities with a designated client
6. Develop a personal "I-Thou" relationship with at least one selected client
7. Discuss with the selected client the effects of hospitalization
8. Discuss retirement with the client
9. Identify the basic human needs that are met through each of the following:
   a. Work
   b. Kinship
   c. Socialization
   d. Environment

Assignment

Following this experience, the student is required to write a paper based on aged client observation. This is due one week after the clinical experience.

Directions

In order to prepare for the paper, first select one client at the senior citizen center and establish an I-Thou relationship. Then complete the following questionnaire based on your experience. This information should be obtained by using third-level communication skills. Do not interview the client.

I. Client Information
   A. Statistics
      Age _____ Sex _____
      Approximate Wt. _____ Approximate Ht. _____
      Marital Status _____ Source of Income _____
   B. Client: Description (In detail)

II. Clinical Experience
   A. State how your selected client meets his or her basic needs (according to Maslow) through each of the following:

      1. Work

      2. Kinship

      3. Socialization

      4. Environment

   B. Summarize your discussion with your client (½ page)

III. Evaluation
   Evaluate your experience at the Center (½ page)

Clinical Focus: Comfort for Pain

I. General Objectives
   Using the nursing process, the student will
   A. Assess the client's needs for comfort.
   B. Establish comfort goals for the client.
   C. Select the best intervention for pain with the client.

II. Specific Objectives
   Building the client's experience, the student will
   A. Assess the client's comfort level and/or pain to discover
      1. Location, onset, duration, history of pain.
      2. Description, characteristics, quality of pain.

3. Factors that increase pain.
4. Factors that reduce pain.
5. Effects on activities of daily living.
6. Effects on relationships.
7. Emotional response to pain.
8. Knowledge and meaning of pain.

B. Discuss with the client his or her experience of pain.

C. List the treatments the client has received or is receiving for analgesic effect.

D. Assess current analgesic therapy.
1. Prepare drug card on medications.
2. Administer drug(s) as needed.
3. Evaluate client's response to medication.

E. Discuss with client the nonpharmacological interventions for pain, including
1. Gate-control theory.
2. Endorphin production.
3. Positioning.
4. Distraction, rhythmic breathing.
5. Hypnosis, guided imagery.

F. Use one of the preceding interventions with the client

G. Evaluate the effectiveness of the intervention

Focus Sheet on Nutritional Assessment

I. General Objectives
Using the nursing process, the student will:
A. Assess client's nutritional status.
B. Assess client's knowledge of basic four food groups.
C. Establish nutrition goals with client.

II. Specific Objectives
Building upon past experiences, the student will:
A. Determine ideal weight for client.
B. Have client record his or her food intake over a 24-hour period (typical).
C. Analyze the above record for deviations from normal.
D. Assess the following:

hair	gums
skin	tongue
teeth	skeletal muscle

E. Examine results of blood and urine studies (serum protein, serum albumin, hemoglobin, plus creatinine).
F. Discuss with client means of maintaining and/or promoting adequate nutrition.

Appendix 6–B

Focus Objectives Relating to Psych-Mental Health Unit

Week 1   Communication

1. Identify situations that facilitate client-nurse interaction.
2. Identify the coping mechanisms utilized by your assigned client.
3. List the effects or potential effects of the client's inability to adequately communicate his or her needs.
4. Identify areas where you may have blocked communication.
5. Identify areas where you may have facilitated communication.

Week 2   Assessment

1. Assess the client's level of adaptation.
2. Identify problems in collaboration with the client.
3. Relate how stress, coping, and adaptation affect the client and his or her family.
4. List behavior patterns of the client.
5. Identify the client's goals related to well-being.

Week 3   Anxiety

1. Assess anxiety with the client.
2. List the effects or potential effects of the client's anxiety.
3. Identify with the client human responses related to anxiety.
4. Identify the effects of the present stress which may affect the client's sexuality.
5. List the nursing measures you used to decrease anxiety.

Week 4   Behavior Reactions

1. Assess the client's feelings regarding his or her behavior.
2. Differentiate between depression and withdrawal.

3. Describe your client's overt behavior.
4. Identify the psychodynamics of your client's behavior.
5. Establish health goals with the client related to his or her behavior reactions.

Leveling of a Specific Topic in Four Courses

Course: Nursing 101

Unit IV: The Nurse, Client, and Family: Oxygen Needs (Exchange and Transport)

Clinical Focus: Oxygen

The student will:

1. Identify stress factors that affect the client's need for oxygen.
2. Identify nursing measures for maintaining oxygen supply.
3. Identify the equipment used to assist clients with oxygen maintenance.
4. Take and record vital signs.
5. Establish goals with client for maintenance of adequate oxygen supply.

Course: Nursing 102

Unit V: The Nurse, Client, and Family: Oxygen Transport Needs

Clinical Focus: Oxygen Transport Needs

The student will:

1. Assess the oxygen transport needs of the client.
2. Discuss with the client the individual factors that affect oxygen transport needs.
3. Identify environmental factors that affect the oxygen transport needs of the client.
4. Assess the client's alteration in fluid volume.
5. Discuss with the client the hazards of fluid imbalance.
6. Discuss with the client the relationship between the medical regimen and oxygen transport needs.

Course: Nursing 201

Unit V: The Nurse, Client, and Family: Oxygen Exchange Needs

Clinical Focus: The Client with Gas Exchange Imbalance

The student will:

1. Assess the client's health status in regard to respiratory function.
2. Assess the client's activity tolerance in relation to his or her oxygen exchange needs.
3. Identify factors in the client's life style that would affect oxygen exchange.
4. Establish health goals related to respiratory function.
5. Describe measures that could be used to prevent or delay progression of the disease process.
6. Assist the client with achievement of established health goals.

Course: Nursing 202

Unit V: The Nurse, Client, and Family: Oxygen Exchange Needs

Clinical Focus: The Client with Inadequate Ventilation

The student will:

1. Assess alterations in airway patency with the client.
2. Complete a detailed assessment of the client's respirations by ear and stethoscope, noting rate, depth, and sound.
3. Listen to breath sounds of the client, evaluating the anterior, lateral, chest apices (posterior), midzones, and bases of lungs.
4. Describe your client's breath sounds.
5. List the effects or potential effects of the client's stress on oxygen exchange.
6. List the factors related to the client that may increase the incidence of problems with oxygen exchange.
7. List the nursing measures you used to increase oxygen to the tissues.
8. Evaluate the success of the interventions with the client.

Appendix 6–D

Contractual Agreement (Agency)

THIS AGREEMENT made and dated as of the _____ day of _____, 19__, by and between _____, hereinafter referred to as

(Name of Nursing College)

"COLLEGE," an institution of higher education having its principal place of operation in the United States of America,

and

_____

(Name of Hospital)

_____

hereinafter called "HOSPITAL."

WITNESSETH, in consideration of the agreements hereinafter contained and other good and valuable considerations, not to include any monetary payment by either party to the other, it is mutually agreed as follows:

COLLEGE does, hereby agree to

1. Provide instructors for teaching and supervising nursing students assigned to the hospital for clinical experience,
2. Have responsibility for planning the schedule of student assignments and making all individual assignments in cooperation with the supervisor and/or charge nurse in the Hospital department(s) used for student experience. (The College expects the selected learning experiences to remain unchanged unless a client's condition demands reassignment. The College will notify the charge nurse and/or supervisor two days prior to any change in schedule necessitated by academic requirements),

131

3. Assume responsibility for College faculty and students complying with all the rules and regulations of the Hospital insofar as they pertain to the activities of both while in the Hospital,
4. Impress upon the instructors and the students their obligation to respect the confidentiality of all records and information that may come to them with regard to the clients' and hospital records,
5. Assume responsibility for nursing faculty and nursing students of the College nursing program carrying professional liability insurance while participating in teaching and learning experiences provided by the Hospital,
6. Assume responsibility for nursing faculty and students providing their own medical care, except in emergencies while on duty in the Hospital,
7. Provide orientation of all levels of nursing service personnel to the philosophy and objectives of the College's associate-degree nursing program,
8. Provide opportunity for nursing service personnel to attend pre- and post-conference sessions of nursing student groups,
9. Specify requirements regarding wearing apparel for nursing students and nursing faculty when on duty in the Hospital.

HOSPITAL does hereby agree to
1. Make available the clinical facilities for student experience, including the necessary equipment and supplies for giving nursing care,
2. Provide
   a. Facilities for change of attire for faculty and students,
   b. Facilities for conference and/or class,
   c. Cafeteria or snack bar services when clinical assignments require it, at the expense of individual faculty member or nursing student,
   d. Orientation and instruction for College faculty relative to the administrative policies and new equipment installed or purchased by the Hospital for patient care or treatment,
3. Make the professional libraries available to the nursing faculty and nursing students,
4. Provide the emergency treatment for any student and/or faculty member at his or her expense if injured during time he or she is in the clinical area,
5. Afford to the nursing faculty and nursing students the privilege of attending professional meetings held at the hospital that would be advantageous to their professional growth,
6. Ensure the cooperation of other agencies using the same facilities for student assignments.

This agreement between COLLEGE and HOSPITAL will be renewed yearly, unless either party notifies the other in writing sixty (60) days before cancellation. No changes or modifications in any and/or all of its provisions shall be binding unless made in writing and signed by the parties. In witness whereof, and intending to be legally bound hereby, the parties hereto have duly executed this agreement.

FOR THE COLLEGE

By _____

Date _____

FOR THE HOSPITAL

By _____

President, Board of Directors

Attested By _____

_____

Date _____

Contractual Agreement (Preceptor/Mentor)

Clarion University of Pennsylvania
Baccalaureate of Science in Nursing

Preceptor/Mentor Agreement

The purpose of this Agreement is to obtain the mutual cooperation of _____
_____ and Clarion University in the provision of
(Preceptor/Mentor)
health care experiences for registered nurse students enrolled in the Baccalaureate
of Science in Nursing Program at the University's Venango Campus.

A. The Preceptor/Mentor agrees to:
1. Participate in an introductory meeting to establish a mutual plan of activity
   which enables the student to meet the course objectives;
2. Develop a plan of action with the student to meet his/her personal objectives within the realities of the practice setting;
3. Plan with the student for experiences which provide for a progression from
   participant observation (if required) toward responsible professional practice;
4. Assist the student to select experiences that facilitate learning;
5. Participate in an exit meeting with the student to review the attainment of
   personal and course objectives;
6. Participate in the evaluation of the student's performance.

B. Clarion University through its Baccalaureate of Science in Nursing Program
   agrees to:
1. Ensure that all BSN students hold certificate of appropriate liability insurance covering all nursing activities;
2. Provide the preceptor/mentor with course objectives prior to the experience;

3. Maintain a contract with the agency for the provision of health care experiences;
4. Obtain written approval for a preceptor/mentor to work with the student while he/she is assigned to the agency;
5. Monitor student activities while in the agency.

C. The Baccalaureate of Science in Nursing student agrees to:
  1. Arrange an introductory meeting with the preceptor/mentor concerning the learning experience;
  2. Provide personal objectives at the introductory meeting;
  3. Arrange with the preceptor/mentor appropriate learning experiences;
  4. Be responsible for his/her learning experiences;
  5. Report to the agency preceptor/mentor prior to each learning experience unless other arrangements have been made;
  6. Be accountable for his/her own nursing actions while in the health agency;
  7. Respect the confidentiality of all information with regard to the client's and agency records;
  8. Arrange an exit meeting to review attainment of personal and course objectives.

The following signatures acknowledge this arrangement and the content within.

_____   _____
Faculty   Date

_____   _____
Preceptor/Mentor   Date

_____   _____
Student   Date

_____

Reprinted with permission of Clarion University of Pennsylvania School of Nursing.

Chapter 7

The Nursing Process and Clinical Instruction

The 1970s brought a heightening of awareness of professional autonomy and accountability to nursing, as nurses examined and questioned previously accepted practices. The current nurse practice acts of most states reflect this trend by their inclusion of the nursing process in the definition of nursing.

The steps of the nursing process (Exhibit 7–1) continuously affect each other and affect validation. Validation, or checking the validity of the process, is mandatory if one subscribes to individual autonomy. Historically, the health care delivery system was governed paternalistically with the we-know-what-is-best-for-you philosophy. Though still evident today, because of present-day consumerism and many determined health care providers, this philosophy is weakening. The beliefs about the individuality of human beings, the environment, and nursing stated in Chapter 1 reflect a new philosophy.

The profession's acknowledgment of the nursing process as a vehicle for operationalizing professional nursing is evidenced by its universal inclusion in curriculum frameworks. Since the nursing process is singled out as the foundation of nursing practice, it is imperative that this strategy be taught and its use encouraged throughout the educational program. The introduction of the nursing process usually occurs in the first nursing course whether a clinical experience is included or not. In programs that omit clinical experience from the initial course, the classroom educator must be creative in offering the student opportunities to apply theoretical knowledge.

Opportunities for teaching and learning the nursing process must be provided throughout the program. Faculty must be committed to the nursing process as a primary focus of the program if it is included as a horizontal curriculum theme. The classroom educator should coordinate the student's learning activities with those utilized by clinical faculty. Faculty, unfortunately, often view the coordination of clinical and classroom teaching activities as an infringement on academic freedom and personal creativity.

Exhibit 7–1 The Nursing Process

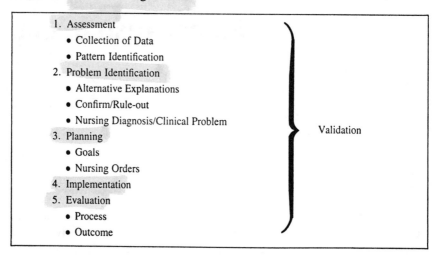

1. Assessment
   - Collection of Data
   - Pattern Identification
2. Problem Identification
   - Alternative Explanations
   - Confirm/Rule-out
   - Nursing Diagnosis/Clinical Problem
3. Planning
   - Goals
   - Nursing Orders
4. Implementation
5. Evaluation
   - Process
   - Outcome

Validation

This infringement may indeed be real; the possibility should be investigated by the appropriate individuals. In most instances, however, the cries of injustice mask teacher ineptness and professional insecurities. If the faculty has identified certain concepts as critical for nursing practice, then these concepts must be internalized and taught by all members of the faculty. Every student must have the opportunity to learn the concepts.

It is important that students be exposed to the belief that the nursing process is dynamic and vital to professional practice. Its value to improving client care should be emphasized rather than its value for rating learner performance. It is the core of nursing practice, a set of skills in which graduating students should be experts and on which the expertise and efficiency of nursing interventions are ultimately dependent. Professional nurses with a sound background in the nursing process should have the expertise to practice safely and competently in most settings.

STRATEGIES FOR TEACHING ASSESSMENT

Assessment, the initial phase of the nursing process, is the deliberate and systematic collection of data to determine clients' current health status and to evaluate their present and past coping patterns. Data is obtained by:

- interview
- physical examination

- observation
- review of records and diagnostic reports
- collaboration (colleagues, clients)

Since interviewing skills are vital to accurate assessments, course content addressing communication theory and skills should precede content on nursing process (see Chapter 8). Students must be given specific opportunities to practice communication techniques.

Even though beginning students have a limited nursing knowledge base, they are frequently required to acquire complete data on their clients. Without stored patterns of nursing knowledge, students cannot assign meaning to the data and thus must feel bombarded with copious amounts of irrelevant pieces of information.

Instead of having students acquire a complete data base, the clinical focus objectives could be structured to provide them with a limited assessment focus. The learners would begin with assessing areas that are familiar to them even without a nursing background, e.g., nutrition, sleep, elimination, skin, vital signs, mobility. Using classroom theory, the students would be expected to gather selected data and to make broad judgments (conclusions) about the data. Thus, they may find a client has inadequate diet, excessive sleep disturbance, good skin integrity.

These students would be expected to care plan only on selected problems. In the next clinical course, the students will be directed with clinical focus objectives to assess for situations they are presently learning. Level II students would be expected to assess and identify the health status related to the theory content presently being studied, e.g., respiratory function, sexuality-sexual function, coping patterns. Of course, the students would also be assessing those areas learned in the level I course. Levels III and IV students will be increasing their stored nursing knowledge and continually adding this theory to their clinical practice. The teaching/learning of the nursing process is a deliberate systematic plan where the learner is guided to eventual spontaneous clinical use. Exhibit 7–2 illustrates the leveling of clinical objectives through four nursing courses.

The Nursing Data Base

The nursing data base is composed of data collected by the student in order to begin to determine patterns, strengths, and alterations. Students will make assessments regarding health status and possible nursing diagnoses. They will also have a responsibility to assess the client in the biomedical realm. If the client has a

Exhibit 7–2 Clinical Objectives and the Nursing Process

At the conclusion of the course, the learner will be able to

Level I:

- collect data in selected functional health patterns—nutrition, elimination, mobility, sleep, rest
- perform physical assessment in selected areas—pulses, blood pressure, respirations, skin, bowel sounds, mouth, appearance of eyes, external ear

Level II:

- collect a complete data base
- perform a complete nursing physical assessment
- demonstrate the use of the nursing process in selected situations on paper

Level III:

- demonstrate the use of the nursing process in selected situations in practice

Level IV:

- demonstrate the use of the nursing process in a variety of clinical situations

pathophysiological process such as diabetes mellitus, students will also ask additional questions such as:

- How is the disease managed? (insulin, oral hypoglycemics, diet)
- Is there evidence of complications? (retinal, renal, vascular)

As nurses acquire more clinical knowledge, the depth and quality of their assessments will improve.

If the learner or the nurse is expected to generate nursing diagnoses from the data base, the educator needs to determine whether the questions will gather data to assist the learner in identifying actual, potential, or possible nursing diagnoses. Are there questions that would elicit information concerning patterns, for example, with regard to coping, relationships, parenting, spirituality?

Physical Assessment

A current trend in nursing education is to teach physical diagnosis. Nursing educators must examine the rationale behind this trend, asking themselves what the general nurse can do with the information acquired as the result of advanced diagnostic skills. If the answer is only "Report the findings to the physician," then perhaps nursing has drifted into the practice of medicine. This is not meant to deprecate the advanced skills of nurses in primary practice who are responsible for physical assessments, screening, and treatment.

Teaching general students how to palpate for enlarged livers or how to use an ophthalmoscope is not in itself inappropriate but becomes so when it means sacrificing the learning of assessment skills crucial for the general nurse. Teaching to differentiate between heart sounds and murmurs but not the palpitation of the location of peripheral pulses may necessitate a reevaluation of curriculum objectives. The nurse generalist must be able to assess signs of increased intracranial pressure but should not be asked to learn an entire neurological assessment. The practice of physical assessment for diagnosing pathophysiology should be left to the experts. The practice of nursing diagnosis for the purpose of assessing human responses should be the primary focus of the generic education of the nurse. In-service educators can use a checklist to determine if new employees possess the critical assessment skills. If they are deficient in any area, several alternatives are available.

Exhibit 7–3 illustrates the physical assessment skills in which nurses should be proficient. Physical diagnosis by nurses should have a nursing focus unless the nurse is practicing beyond a generalist's scope as a clinical specialist or a nurse practitioner.

Cues and Inferences

Teaching the assessment component is begun by assisting students to differentiate between cues and information (see Exhibit 7–4). The ability to make this distinction is of paramount importance because inferences based on few cues or none can sometimes result in erroneous and injurious care. Consider the following case:

> A 72-year-old woman is hospitalized complaining of abdominal pain. All diagnostic tests prove negative. The staff infer that her pain is psychosomatic because of the negative studies. The staff should have gathered more cues to support their inference. Instead, the woman suffered alone for one week until her intestinal obstruction was diagnosed.

The educator must stress the importance of gathering cues. Students should be asked to assess the client and then review cues with the instructor. Initially, the focus of assessment should be limited according to clinical objectives, say to skin, pain, or coping patterns. Giving a beginning student an entire assessment form to

Exhibit 7–3 Physical Assessment by Nurse Generalists

Physical System	Criteria
Sensory-Perceptual	Mental status
	Vision and appearance of eyes
	Hearing
	Touch
	Taste and smell
Skin	Condition (color, turgor, character)
	Lesions
	Edema
	Hair distribution
Respiratory	Rate, character
	Breath sounds
	Cough
Cardiovascular	Pulses (rate, quality, rhythm)
	Apical Radial
	Carotid Dorsalis pedis
	Brachial Posterior tibial
	Femoral
	Blood pressure
	Circulation (mucous membranes, nail beds)
Neurological	Pupillary reactions
	Orientation
	Level of consciousness
	Grasp strength
Gastrointestinal	Mouth, gums, teeth, and tongue (color, condition)
	Gag reflex
	Bowel sounds
	Presence of distention, impaction, hemorrhoids (external)
Genitourinary	Lesions
	Presence of retention
	Discharge (vaginal, urethral)
	Uterine response (pregnancy, postpartum)
Musculoskeletal	Muscle tone, strength
	Gait, stability
	Range of motion

complete would be as inappropriate as requiring a student to present a thesis in a beginning research course.

After cues are identified, inferences can be made. With each inference made, the student should be asked: How do you know that? This is a helpful strategy for eliminating inferences based on shallow or nonexistent cues. After examining the cues the student may decide that more data are needed to make a valid inference.

Cues as well as inferences must be validated with the client. From a particular set of cues depression may be inferred. The nurse needs to explore this possibility

Exhibit 7-4 Cues and Inferences in Client Assessment

- A cue about the client is information that one acquires by seeing, touching, tasting, hearing, or smelling. Sources of cues are the client (primarily), the client's significant others (secondarily), and diagnostic tests.
- An inference is the interpretation of the data of the cue. Interpretation is based on one's knowledge, values, and experiences.[1]

Examples

Cue	Inference
Hgb. 9.1	Abnormal
Fruity breath	Acidotic
Height 5'1", weight 210 lb.	Obesity

---

with the client. Inferences not confirmed or those where more data are needed should be labeled questionable. Students should be encouraged to follow their hunches but always to be seeking validation.

Values Clarification

Much has been written on values clarification and the effects of personal values on performance. Including values clarification in course content on the nursing process will assist the student to recognize these effects. The following short exercise might be used by students and practicing nurses to increase their awareness of certain beliefs and values and their implications for care:

Write adjectives and nouns to describe the following:

Obese female
Alcoholic
Unmarried 16-year-old mother-to-be

After completing the exercise, students should discuss what they have written down. The instructor must help the students to explore their feelings as reflected by the words they chose and help them recognize how these feelings can affect the care they provide.

Values clarification exercises can be integrated into the curriculum to assist the learners with identification of their own feelings and prejudices. Certain sensitive issues or subjects provide excellent topics: death and dying, addiction, sexuality, domestic violence, abortion, and disabilities. Exhibit 7–5 is an example of a values clarification exercise on disabilities that students would complete prior to a group discussion.

Exhibit 7–5 Values Clarification Exercise

---

1. You are standing in a crowded bus. Put 1 next to the person you would most like to stand next to and continue until number 6 is given to the person you would least like to stand next to.

   _____ Blind
   _____ Body odor
   _____ Very obese
   _____ Spastic muscular dystrophy
   _____ Amputated arm
   _____ Severely burn-scarred face

2. Check which of the following are associated with carelessness and/or bad character.

   _____ Bad breath
   _____ Body odor
   _____ Amputation
   _____ Obesity (20 percent over ideal weight)

3. Finish each statement with your spontaneous thoughts.
   a. When I see a blind person I _____

   _____

   b. To me, getting around in a wheelchair _____

   _____

   c. If I had cancer of the tongue, _____

   _____

4. Rank the disability or physical difference you would feel most *distressed* to have as 1 and continue until 6 are ranked.

   _____ Obesity
   _____ Deaf
   _____ Paralyzed legs
   _____ Bad scar on face
   _____ Colostomy
   _____ Laryngectomy

5. Interview a person with a physical difference (blind, deaf, obese, paralyzed, scarred, etc.).
   a. Ask the person how people respond to his or her physical difference.
   b. Ask the person how he or she would like people to respond.

Unfortunately, in the process of integrating nursing into their lives, students acquire the erroneous belief that to be a good professional nurse, one must be something less than human: "The educational and practice situations in nursing often prevent or at best discourage the nurse from being too sensitive to or getting too involved with another's feelings."[2] The authors of a 1959 nursing text observed that nurses need to "humor" difficult patients[3] and "must learn often with difficulty to turn the other cheek."[4] Historically, students of nursing were taught that they must always put aside their feelings in order to nurse, whereas in reality you cannot actualize nursing if you are devoid of feelings. Such an attitude often resulted in the suppression of hostility, which would surface in some other aspect of a nurse's professional life.

There are times when one cannot nurse a client effectively. A prudent nurse will recognize the signs, for first and foremost nurses are human beings. Nurses who deny their humanity will soon acquire the characteristics so often used to describe nurses as cold, insensitive, frustrated, and uncaring.

Teaching/Learning Strategies

Assessment skills can be taught by various techniques limited in variety only by the creativity of the faculty. A few examples are the use of audiovisuals, programmed instruction, and independent study. Classroom instruction can be combined effectively with independent study as in the following illustration:

Students are assigned to view a videotape of an instructor performing a skin assessment. This is supplemented with an assigned reading. Students each must then perform a skin assessment on three acquaintances, selecting one person from each of three age groups: birth to 18 months, 40–65, and 66–80. Supplementing their assessment would be discussions to assist the students in comparing and contrasting age-related and ethnic skin differences. This approach can be expanded to other assessment tools. Faculty, however, need to determine when a practice laboratory session may be needed to supplement the independent study, as for respiratory assessments.

The nursing history is a systematic interview of a newly admitted client by a professional nurse for the purpose of acquiring data to provide criteria for diagnosis and intervention. The nursing history should focus on assessing the individual's response to life processes, problems, deviation from health, activities of daily living, and interactions.

The nursing history form should be sufficiently structured to afford the student or new graduate some ease in data collection. As the beginner gains expertise in interviewing, the form can be relegated to reference status.

Before being assigned a complete nursing history, the student should have the opportunity to practice interviewing skills and assessment in selected areas of the form. This provides the students with successful achievement of assessment skills before being required to have mastered the completed admission history. The instructor can assign assessment in the clinical setting with related form sheets or

Exhibit 7–6 Focus Sheet on Nutritional Assessment

I. General Objectives

Using the nursing process the student will
A. Assess the client's nutritional status
B. Assess the client's knowledge of the four basic food groups
C. Establish nutrition goals with the client

II. Specific Objectives

Building upon past experiences, the student will
A. Determine ideal weight for the client
B. Discuss with the client his or her food intake over a typical 24-hour period
C. Analyze this record for deviations from normal
D. Assess the following
Hair	Gums
Skin	Tongue
Teeth	Skeletal muscle
E. Examine results of blood and urine studies (serum protein, serum albumin, hemoglobin, plus creatinine)
F. Discuss with the client means of maintaining or promoting adequate nutrition

---

can have the students do an independent study on selected friends or family members as clients. Exhibit 7–6 illustrates the kind of focus sheet that can be used for either task.

A videotape of the instructor obtaining data by using a nursing history form would provide students with an opportunity to watch an interview and physical assessment. The tape should also show that the interview depends upon the style and nature of the participants as well as the subject matter being discussed.

If several varieties of forms are used, then several videotapes are needed. Audiotape cassettes are an alternative but do not allow students to observe the physical assessment. Viewing a videotape or listening to an audio cassette gives students some familiarity with interviewing prior to actually trying it. They will initially probably parrot the instructor's style and words for security. Faculty cannot expect students to develop their own individual styles until they are comfortable with interviewing.

After students successfully perform limited data collection assignments, they can progress to the comprehensive nursing history. This assessment can be accomplished during the preclinical experience described previously. If this experience is omitted in the program, the following alternative is suggested: Reserve 45 minutes to one hour of afternoon clinical time during which students will not be responsible for client care. Assign each student to a new admission for the purpose of conducting the nursing interview. New admissions are most desirable because the student has an opportunity to acquire data uninfluenced by previously recorded information. If admission assessments are not possible on the clinical unit, arrangements can be made with the agency to select clients from other units. It is beneficial for students to be assigned to the same client the following day if possible, thus allowing continued assessment, evaluation, and refinement of the history.

New staff nurses should be introduced to assessment and nursing history procedures during orientation. A classroom session should be followed by application on their assigned units. The new employee's success or failure with the nursing history will dictate how much concentrated learning is needed. Care planning can be better facilitated if assignments are consistent for five to seven days and can be most successful if primary nursing is utilized.

The students and the new employee should be required to return to the instructor within two days or so for an analysis of the data collected. The student should be asked what cues were collected and what inferences were derived. Evidence of validation should be expected. Students may also be asked to evaluate their own skills as interviewers. As the student approaches mastery, this exercise need not be a written requirement. The educator can reinforce the process by asking students to collect cues in particular situations. For example, if a student states: "My client's blood pressure is high," the student has made an inference, but one based on a single blood pressure reading. The student should be required to review the chart to collect data on past readings and to examine factors that may contribute to a high reading before making another inference. After successfully completing this stage, the student can progress to problem identification.

STRATEGIES FOR TEACHING PROBLEM IDENTIFICATION

Problem identification, the second component of the nursing process, incorporates intellectual activities that focus on identifying interaction patterns, validating the findings, and evolving a statement about the health status of the individual. The term *nursing diagnosis* is frequently used in place of *problem identification* as the second step in the nursing process.[5] *Nursing diagnosis* will be used exclusively in this book to describe a classification system of diagnostic labels, not the process of analysis of data.

Problem identification or the cognitive analysis of data for possible patterns is very difficult to teach and to learn because the learner must have access to stored patterns of clinical knowledge. Skilled clinical knowledge is a combination of theoretical understanding and practice knowledge. Skilled clinical knowledge occurs after exposure to many practical situations. It develops the nurse's ability to single out relevant information from irrelevant and assigns qualitative characteristics to data because of clinical expertise.[6]

Students and new graduates are often laden with theoretical knowledge but lack clinical skills. Thus the new clinician strives to acquire more clinical skills and as a result the acquisition of theoretical knowledge may become secondary. The measure of an expert professional is one who encompasses both theoretical and clinical learning as a lifelong pursuit and responsibility. Figure 7–1 is a schematic diagram depicting the acquisition of clinical knowledge. The educator can systematically assist the learner to acquire skilled clinical knowledge by

- providing learners access to varied clinical experiences either as individuals or in group conferences
- requiring the learner to generate several possible explanations for data even when one explanation seems to be the correct one
- sharing with the learner one's own rich skilled clinical knowledge

---

Figure 7–1 Acquisition of Skilled Clinical Knowledge

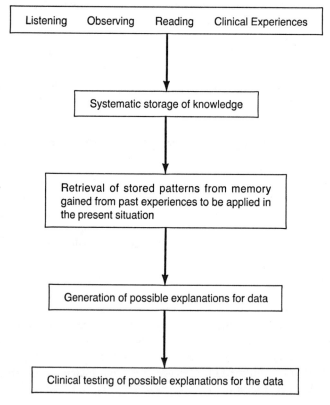

Discussions of possible explanations for data can be done informally on the clinical unit with an actual situation or formally in the classroom using case studies. The learner could be asked to generate possible explanations for data using a decision-tree format.

72-year-old woman with disorientation in time, place

medications   hypoxia   environmental   sleep disruption   metabolic imbalances

The above represents some possible explanations for the data. Without the cultivation of possible explanations for the disorientation, the learner may unfairly or wrongly label the condition as senility. One can experiment with this strategy also, for example, by changing the age from 72 to 42, and evaluate if the responses take on another focus.

DEFINING THE PROBLEM

After the data has been analyzed and alternative explanations tested and ruled out, one of the following conclusions will represent the outcome for grouped data:[7]

- no problem evident at this time; no health promotion activities needed
- no problem evident at this time; health promotion activities indicated
- actual, potential, possible clinical problems
- actual, potential, possible nursing diagnoses

Nursing Diagnosis Versus Clinical Collaborative Problems

In 1973 the North American Nursing Diagnosis Association (formerly The National Group for the Classification of Nursing Diagnosis) was organized to develop and classify nursing diagnosis for clinical testing. The purpose of these classifying activities is to identify and structure nursing phenomena and nursing's unique domain. Nurses have little difficulty in implementing the medical regimen or identifying problems that are directly related to medical diagnoses. The use of nursing diagnoses permits the nurse to go beyond the medical model and identify those problems that may or may not be related to medical diagnoses. For nursing to become a full profession, it must develop and accept a classification system that will represent nursing's independent accountable domain.

Nurses intervene with two types of diagnoses (problems, health states). The first are those situations in which the nurse collaborates with other members of the health team to treat. Nurses do not prescribe the primary treatments for these situations but are actively involved in the treatment regimen and do make independent decisions in these situations. These situations are called clinical problems.[8] For example, an individual in a coronary intensive care unit is monitored for potential arrhythmias. It is the nurse's responsibility to diagnose and treat arrhythmias. However, the treatment of the arrhythmia has been ordered by the physician, not the nurse.

The second type of clinical situation involves those problems or health states wherein the nurse can legally prescribe the primary interventions for the situation. These conditions are labeled with nursing diagnostic terminology.

In documentation, as in care plans, clinical problems can be labeled with the appropriate terminology, e.g., hypovolemia (post-op), hyperglycemia. The nurse should not be placing medical diagnoses on nursing care plans. Rather the individual's response to the medical diagnosis and/or treatments is assessed and these responses are recorded as nursing diagnoses or clinical problems. Exhibit 7–7 lists examples of clinical problems.

The key to differentiating clinical problems from nursing diagnoses is whether the nurse can legally order the majority or primary of the interventions to treat the problem. This framework recognizes that collaborative interventions are legitimate, expert responsibilities of nurses and should not require nursing diagnostic terminology to make them creditable or acceptable for a nursing care plan.

Nursing diagnosis has acquired a risky priority, seemingly reducing to unimportance the other problems that nurses are responsible for, monitoring and treating. Expert clinical nurses need to focus on pathophysiology in their assessments as well as functional health patterns. The practice setting of the nurse and/or the condition of the client will determine what focus the assessment and interventions will take.

The educator should reevaluate the practice of requiring students to care plan only with nursing diagnoses. This policy either forces students to make up terminology, to rewrite the clinical problem in nursing diagnosis terminology or encourages the omission of these problems on care plans. If care plans are to be restricted for nursing diagnoses only, the student must be provided with additional forms in order to record the clinical problems and associated interventions.

It is important that all faculty in a school be consistent in their definitions and terminology related to nursing diagnosis. It is very frustrating and unfair to the students when one instructor rejects terms previously accepted by another. Students benefit from having a list of accepted diagnoses; if the faculty approve, the national list shown in Exhibit 7–8 is recommended.

Exhibit 7–7 Examples of Clinical Problems

- potential for hypoglycemia
- potential complications of mechanical ventilation
- potential for increased intracranial pressure
- potential complications of cardiac arrhythmias

Students can label the diagnosis as actual, potential, or possible. A possible nursing diagnosis is a condition that may exist for which more data must be gathered to make certain. A potential diagnosis is a problem that may occur if certain nursing actions are not initiated to prevent it. Students should be cautioned that whenever possible a nursing diagnosis must be validated with the client to be an actual diagnosis. If the client does not accept it as a problem or the nurse cannot alleviate, reduce, or prevent the outcome, then the nursing diagnosis is not legitimate.

The following is an example of an erroneous nursing diagnosis resulting from the incongruent values of the nurse and the client:

A heavy smoker is told by his physician after his second myocardial infarction to quit smoking. The man continues to smoke. The student's nursing diagnosis is "noncompliance."

The student needs to ask: How do I know that? What are the cues? If the client is not well informed about the relation between smoking and cardiovascular function, then the diagnosis may be "Knowledge deficit related to the effects of smoking on cardiovascular function." However, if the client is well informed about the relation of smoking to vasoconstriction, then that diagnosis is also erroneous. If the philosophy of freedom of choice on the part of the client is supported by the nurse, the diagnosis of noncompliance is unacceptable. If a client chooses not to participate in the prescribed health care regimen the problem may lie not with the client but with the prescription and the prescribers. Thus the client's nursing diagnosis should not be related to his continued smoking.

It is important that students and graduates derive nursing diagnoses from data collected by nurses and not be influenced by the medical diagnosis and chart information. The latter can support a nursing diagnosis but cannot serve as the only criteria for its derivation. A creative educator may incorporate the following exercise to prevent students from being strongly influenced by medical data: The student is deliberately not informed of the medical diagnosis and chart information prior to obtaining the nursing history and performing the physical assessment. The

Exhibit 7–8 Accepted Nursing Diagnoses List (1982)

Activity Intolerance

Airway Clearance, Ineffective

Anxiety

Bowel Elimination, Alteration in:
Constipation

Bowel Elimination, Alteration in: Diarrhea

Bowel Elimination, Alteration in:
Incontinence

Breathing Patterns, Ineffective

Cardiac Output, Alterations in: Decreased

Comfort, Alterations in: Pain

Communication, Impaired Verbal

Coping, Ineffective Individual

*Coping, Ineffective Family: Compromised

Coping, Ineffective Family: Disabling

Coping, Family: Potential for Growth

Diversional Activity, Deficit

Family Processes, Alteration in

Fear

Fluid Volume Deficit

Fluid Volume Deficit, Potential

Fluid Volume, Excess

Gas Exchange, Impaired

Grieving, Anticipatory

Grieving, Dysfunctional

Health Maintenance, Alteration in

Home Maintenance Management,
Impaired

*Infection, Potential for

Injury, Potential for

Knowledge Deficit (specify)

Mobility, Impaired Physical

Non-compliance (specify)

Nutrition, Alternation in: Less than body
requirements

Nutrition, Alteration in: More than body
requirements

Nutrition, Alteration in: Potential for more
than body requirements

Oral Mucous Membrane, Alteration in

Parenting, Alteration in: Actual, Potential

Powerlessness

Rape-Trauma Syndrome

Respiratory Function, Alteration in

Self-Care Deficit:
feeding
bathing/hygiene
dressing/grooming
toileting

Self-Concept, Disturbance in

Sensory Perceptual Alteration:
visual
auditory
kinesthetic
gustatory
tactile
olfactory

Sexual Dysfunction

Skin Integrity, Impairment, Actual

Skin Integrity, Impairment, Potential

Sleep Pattern, Disturbance

*Social Interactions, Impaired

Social Isolation

Spiritual Distress

Thought Processes, Alterations in

Tissue perfusion, Alteration in:
cerebral
cardiopulmonary
renal
gastrointestinal
peripheral

Urinary Elimination, Alteration in Patterns
of

Violence, Potential for

*These diagnoses have been added from *Handbook of Nursing Diagnoses*, by L.J. Carpenito, J.B. Lippincott, 1984.

student is directed to utilize assessment skills to identify data pertinent to nursing. After the assessment the student will cite inferences and then can review the chart.

Inservice educators may have more difficulty with graduate and experienced nurses relying on medical diagnoses. Unfortunately, many nurses focus on identifying clinical data that are relevant primarily to the physician, rather than data relevant to nursing care. Part of nursing practice is the collection of data for the sole purpose of reporting it to the physicians. However, some of this data collection is repeated by the physician. Repetition should be avoided in an effort to save the nurse time needed to collect data relevant to the nurse's independent practice.

As students become more skilled in deriving nursing diagnoses they should be encouraged to evolve new diagnostic categories. If nursing is going to develop a taxonomy of diagnoses, then students of the profession should be encouraged to participate in the process of generating new categories. Appendix 7–A lists guidelines adapted from the North American Nursing Diagnosis Association. This system is especially beneficial for practicing nurses who find the approved list limiting. Staff development departments can draw up their own in-agency lists to supplement the national list, with the goal of submitting new diagnostic categories to the National Association.

Strategies for Teaching Nursing Diagnosis

The educator can utilize several techniques to teach students about nursing diagnosis. Some are:

- Giving a didactic presentation on the nursing process with content on nursing diagnosis
- Assigning readings
- Adding nursing diagnoses to nursing courses, beginning with the simple and advancing to the more complex diagnoses (see Exhibit 7–9)
- Formulating clinical focus objectives for each nursing diagnosis category to direct the learner to specific assessment and implementation activities (see Exhibit 7–10)

Just as students are introduced to each nursing diagnosis in the curriculum, agency educators can introduce staff nurses to the diagnostic categories with specific strategies. Staff nurses will need an organized inservice program on the concept of nursing diagnosis and on the categories. After this initial information exchange, each nursing unit can be provided with the list of accepted nursing diagnoses, their defining characteristics, and etiological/contributing factors. Merely posting a list of nursing diagnoses on units is unsatisfactory.

Exhibit 7–9 Distribution of Nursing Diagnoses in a Nursing Curriculum

---

NURSING 101
  Self-Care Deficits
  Impairment of Skin Integrity
  Alteration of Bowel Elimination
  Alteration in Nutrition
  Alteration in Comfort
  Diversional Activity Deficit
  Potential for Injury

NURSING 102
  Activity Intolerance
  Alteration in Respiratory Function
  Alteration in Cardiac Output
  Fluid Volume (excess, deficit)
  Impaired Physical Mobility
  Alterations in Oral Mucous Membrane
  Health Maintenance, Alteration in
  Sensory Perceptual Alterations
  Sleep Pattern Disturbance
  Urinary Elimination, Alteration in patterns of

NURSING 201
  Impaired Verbal Communication
  Anxiety
  Coping, Ineffective Individual
  Coping, Ineffective Family
  Family Processes, Alteration in
  Fear
  Knowledge Deficit
  Parenting, Alteration in
  Spiritual Distress
  Thought Processes, Alteration in
  Violence, Potential for

NURSING 202
  Grieving
  Home Maintenance Management, Impaired
  Non-compliance
  Powerlessness
  Rape-Trauma Syndrome
  Self-Concept, Disturbance in
  Sexual Dysfunction
  Social Isolation

Exhibit 7–10 Clinical Focus Objectives for Spiritual Distress

---

I. General Objectives
Using the nursing process, the student will:
A. Assess the client's spiritual dimension
B. Formulate an actual, potential, or possible nursing diagnosis of spiritual distress if indicated
II. Specific Objectives
The student will:
A. Prior to the experience, read:
1. Carpenito, L.J., "Spiritual Distress," pp. 451–466, in *Nursing Diagnosis/Application to Clinical Practice* (Philadelphia: J.B. Lippincott, 1983).
2. Shannon, M., "Spiritual Needs and Nursing Responsibility," *Imprint* 10, no. 12 (1980): 23.
3. Stoll, R.I., "Guidelines for Spiritual Assessment," *American Journal of Nursing* 79 (1979): 1574–1577.
B. Assess the spiritial dimension of an individual. Suggested questions:
1. "Is religion or God important to you?" If answer is yes, "To what religion do you belong?" or "In what do you believe?" If no, "Do you find a source of strength or meaning in another area?"
2. "What effect do you expect your illness (hospitalization) to have on your spiritual practices or beliefs?"
3. "Are there any religious books (statues, medals, services, places) that are especially important to you?"
4. "Do you have a special religious leader (priest, pastor, rabbi)?"
5. "How can I help you maintain your spiritual strength during this illness (hospitalization)?" (e.g., contact spiritual leader, provide privacy at special times, request reading materials)
C. Observe for
1. The presence of religious or spiritual articles (clothing, medals, texts)
2. Visits from religious leader
3. Visits to religious place of worship (chapel)
4. Requests for spiritual counseling or assistance
5. The response to interview on spiritual needs (anxiety, doubt, anger, depression)
D. Assess for the presence of defining characteristics of spiritual distress:
1. Experiences a disturbance in belief system
    a. questions credibility of belief system
    b. is discouraged
    c. is unable to practice usual religious rituals
    d. has ambivalent feelings (doubts) about beliefs
    e. feels a sense of spiritual emptiness
2. Expresses concern—anger, resentment, fear—with meaning of life, suffering, death
3. Requests spiritual assistance
E. Identify factors that may contribute to spiritual distress in this individual.
Examples:
    a. loss of body part or function
    b. terminal disease
    c. debilitating disease
    d. death or illness of significant other

Exhibit 7–10 continued

> e. embarrassment at practicing spiritual rituals
> f. hospital barriers to practicing spiritual rituals (isolation, confinement to bed or room, intensive care restrictions, trauma)
> g. prescribed medical regimen (surgery, dietary restrictions, medications, medical procedures, e.g., IVs)
> h. conflicts with belief system (abortion, surgery or blood transfusion—when prohibited by religion, pain, divorce)
> i. beliefs opposed by family, peers, health care providers

The staff development department could compile articles and assessment questions on each nursing diagnosis and place them in an envelope labeled with that diagnosis. Every two to four weeks the envelopes (approximately 50) would be rotated from one unit to another. During the time period that the specific nursing diagnosis is on the unit, staff should be encouraged to review the material. Client care conferences during this time period would focus on individuals who have that specific nursing diagnosis. If there are no individuals on the unit with the specific nursing diagnosis, e.g., Rape-Trauma Syndrome, then the unit could:

- assign one nurse to present a case study of a person with the diagnosis
- arrange for an inservice program with a speaker who is familiar with the care of an individual with the diagnosis.

STRATEGIES FOR TEACHING

Planning and Intervention

Care plans are the documentation of three steps in the nursing process—problem identification, planning (goals and interventions), and evaluation. As noted, the learner can be introduced to care planning in stages, beginning with the evaluation of a problem list for a client and progressing to a complete care plan on a client.

Should students be required to write a care plan on every individual they care for? Frequently, the term *care plan* and *case study* are confused. Often students are required to write care plans; however, the finished product resembles a case study. Case studies are valuable teaching/learning strategies but it is unrealistic and unnecessary for students to develop case studies for each client.

Students can be required to generate a complete problem list (actual, potential, possible) on their clients. However, they should be asked to care plan on only a maximum of three problems. The rationale for this strategy is that the care plan will contain the three problem or health status areas that the student will be focusing on that day. The student is specifically accountable for this part of the plan. It is unreasonable for the educator to believe that the student will address the 8–12 problems listed in the care plan on a single day. If students are not expected to intervene in all the problems, then the educators are sending a message to students that it is sufficient to write care plans and not important to implement them. Requiring students to care plan only on limited numbers of problems reflects a more practical, professional approach.

As students progress through the curriculum, they would not repeatedly care plan on routine interventions such as asepsis or safety. (Of course, if the client is at high risk for infection or injury, then care planning on this problem would be appropriate.) Seniors could probably delete the rationale for most of their interventions, unless they are in a newly taught content area, e.g., powerlessness.

Students should progress to care plan only with interventions that are specific to the client or to identify a client who is at high risk to develop a problem. Should a student repeatedly care plan on routine interventions the educator can request that the student not care plan on the client prior to the clinical experience. On the day of the experience the educator can then assist the student in the assessment of data that may previously have been ignored or not known. In certain situations, faculty may be expecting students to identify specific nursing diagnoses for their client which in reality require repetitive nurse-client interactions to assess for or treat. Perhaps students can be directed to assess for the presence by stating the problem as "possible." A possible nursing diagnosis is an indication that the nurse needs additional data to confirm or rule out the diagnosis.

Strategies for Teaching Care Planning

Nursing Diagnoses/Clinical Problems

The identification of the health status or problem statement is probably the most difficult component of the care plan to teach and to learn. If learners are having difficulty evaluating the problem statement, they may skip this column and the goal column and proceed to the intervention column. Most nurses know what they want to do for a client but have difficulty labeling the problem. After the nurse has written the interventions, she/he can go back to the problem column and write the statement.

When writing a nursing diagnosis, students should be encouraged or required to use the accepted terminology from the North American Nursing Association. They should also be encouraged to generate new nursing diagnoses with defining characteristics when the list does not provide a diagnostic category that describes the present situation. Faculty and students should be cautioned when evolving new categories that they are not describing a clinical problem instead of a nursing diagnosis. As discussed earlier in this chapter, nurses intervene with two types of diagnoses (clinical problems and nursing diagnoses), students should not be required to care plan only with nursing diagnoses. This practice forces students to reword collaborative problems as increased intracranial pressure into nursing diagnoses terminology. The implications of this practice can only serve to obstruct the intent to develop a classification system which is to identify the body of knowledge that professional nurses are accountable for.

In order to clearly differentiate a nursing diagnosis from a clinical problem, especially when the student is creatively and appropriately generating new nursing diagnoses, the student should be asked to write after the statement a N Dx or a C.P. Another method is to add a small column on the care plan to record this as:

Date	Problem or Diagnosis	Nsg. Dx/ C.P.	Goals	Plan	Evaluation

After the problem statement has been formulated, the learner should be required to record the assessment data that validated this problem. Some faculty prefer that the student add "as manifested by" to the statement followed by the signs and symptoms. For example:

> Impairment of Skin Integrity:
> Pressure ulcer related to immobility ° to pain as manifested by a 2 cm erythemic area over sacral area and reluctance to change position because of pain.

Since the addition of the signs and symptoms to the problem statement can make for a very lengthy problem statement, an alternative method of validation may prove more useful (see Exhibit 7–11).

In evaluating the quality and accuracy of the nursing diagnosis statement, the educator (and the learner) should consider the following:

1. Is the statement clearly stated?
2. Is the terminology correct?
3. Is there a two-part statement?
4. Does the second part of the statement reflect the specific factors that have or may have contributed to the development of the nursing diagnosis?
5. Is there documentation of validation? (signs and symptoms)

Exhibit 7–11 Validation of Nursing Diagnosis on a Care Plan

Date	Diagnosis
6-5	Impairment of Skin Integrity: Pressure Ulcer related to immobility ° to pain Signs and Symptoms: 2 cm erythemic area over sacral area reluctance to change position because "I have pain."

6. Does the nursing diagnosis statement reflect a situation for which a nurse can order the majority of interventions to treat or prevent?
7. Does the problem list appropriately reflect actual, potential, or possible nursing diagnoses or clinical problems?

Goals

Outcome criteria or client goals are written to identify the desired outcome and to measure the effectiveness of the plan. Goals are formulated with the client or family to:

- maintain the present state of health
- improve the present state of health
- obtain optimal adaption to altered health status
- obtain optimal levels of coping
- prevent complications and disabilities

In evaluating the goals on the student's care plan, the educator should consider the following:

1. Is the goal a client goal or a nursing goal?
2. Is the goal realistic and attainable?
3. Is it measurable? (Can the nurse validate it by seeing or hearing?)
4. Are the verbs measurable ("states," "demonstrates") or not measurable ("knows," "understands," "experiences")?
5. Has the content been clearly specified (how much, when, where)?
6. Can a time for achievement be realistically identified?

Nursing Orders/Interventions

The care plan is the vehicle for communicating to other nurses and auxiliary nursing personnel what interventions have been prescribed by a professional nurse. The plan should be organized according to priorities so as to assist the student in determining what interventions are critical. For the student beginning the transition to graduate nurse, deciding priorities will help ensure that critical interventions are addressed.

A detailed interview and physical assessment is of little value unless the data are analyzed and directions for care specified. The specific directions for prescribing nursing care are given in the nursing order, which has the following components:[9]

1. Date
2. (Directive verb)
3. When, how often, how long
4. What and where
5. Signature

The nursing order directs care to the client on shifts and days when the nurse who prescribed it is not present. If a member of the unit disagrees with an order, it is acceptable to question it. It is not acceptable to ignore it. Very often with additional data, nursing orders need to be updated, discontinued, or revised.

Students may be forced by necessity to use textbooks to supplement their care plans. They must be encouraged to use specificity in writing orders to reflect the individuality of the client. For example, after completing an assessment on an assigned client, the student concludes the following:

Cues	Inferences	Nursing Diagnosis	Nursing Order
Viscid expectorations,	Dehydration	Fluid	Force
Skin turgor,		volume deficit	fluids
Dry oral mucosa,			
COPD			
Urine specific gravity 1.007			

The student must be asked what does *force fluids* mean? How does the nurse evaluate whether the order to force fluids has been accomplished? The student must assess the individual client to determine the specifics of the order. The new nursing order might read

Encourage fluids at least 2000 cc/day

Time	Amount
7–3	800
3–11	800
11–7	400

Likes orange juice, ginger ale, water. Can have coffee and tea as extra fluids, but do not calculate them for the 2000 cc/day.

The writing of nursing orders that reflect the individuality of the client is made easier by continuity of assignments. The more contact a nurse has with a client, the more specific the orders usually are.

In evaluating the nursing orders on the student's care plan, the educator should consider the following:

1. Are the nursing orders clear (what, when, how often, how long, where)?
2. Does the nurse need additional client contact to individualize the nursing orders?
3. Do the nursing orders reflect creativity (thinking, unusual references)?

Evaluation

Evaluation is the final component of the nursing process, but in reality it is an element of each component. The nurse continually evaluates with every nurse-client interaction.

In evaluating the entire plan of care, the student will be directed to consider the following questions for each component:

- Nursing Diagnosis
  1. Does the diagnosis still exist?
  2. Does the potential diagnosis still exist?
  3. Has the possible diagnosis been confirmed or ruled out?
  4. Does a new diagnosis need to be added?
- Goals
  1. Have goals been resolved?
  2. Do goals reflect the present focus of care?
  3. Can more specific modifiers be added?
- Interventions
  1. Are interventions acceptable to the client?
  2. Are interventions specific to the client?
  3. Do interventions provide clear instructions for the nursing staff?

In considering the above questions, the student would then record one of the following decisions in the evaluation column:

- Evaluation
  1. Continue: The diagnosis is still present and the goals and interventions are appropriate.

2. Revised: The diagnosis is still present, but the goals or nursing orders require revision. The revisions are then recorded.
3. Ruled out/confirmed: A possible diagnosis has been confirmed or ruled out by additional data collection. Goals and nursing orders are written if needed.
4. Resolved: A diagnosis has been resolved and that portion of the care plan is discontinued.

Standardized Care Plans

Agencies or units with a client population having similar nursing diagnoses may choose to formulate standardized care plans. Such plans suggest to the nurses specific interventions and obviate time-consuming writing. They do not replace the individualized assessment of the client, however, for nursing diagnoses that are specific to the client rather than to one's clinical or medical diagnosis are still needed. The nurse initiating the care plan will cross out areas of the standardized care plan that do not apply or are contraindicated and add nursing diagnoses pertinent to the client.

Exhibit 7–12 is an example of part of a standardized care plan for a surgical client pre-op. This plan would be preprinted for use on any unit with a client who is to undergo surgery. It would provide nurses with direction and would be signed when done. A standardized care plan for the post-op care of a client undergoing a total hip replacement would direct care common to such clients. Individualized nursing care is not hindered by this process, and in fact the reduction of lengthy writing provides the professional nurse with more time for individualized nursing care. It also assists caregivers who are not expert in this particular care with detailed directions. Exhibit 7–13 represents a section from a standardized care plan for a client undergoing a total hip replacement.

Exhibit 7–12 A Standardized Care Plan for a Surgical Pre-op Client

Nursing Diagnosis	*Nursing Orders*
1. Knowledge deficit related to surgical experience	1a. Verbalize typical post-op course and precautions to prevent dislocation of the hip joint. b. Verbalize other possible complications. c. Have patient read pre-op guide. d. Explore patient's goals.
2. Possible fear related to unknown	2a. Explore fears and feelings. b. Give concrete information when appropriate.

Exhibit 7–13 Section of a Standardized Health Care Plan

Nursing Diagnosis	*Nursing Orders*
Potential impairment of skin integrity related to immobility and incision.	1. Egg crate mattress (use two if body weight is greater than 113.6 kgm). 2. Tilt on nonoperative side and back q2h. Keep head of bed flat when tilted. 3. Skin inspection and back massage with lotion q2h. If area is reddened, refer to procedure manual (re decubitus ulcer care). 4. Instruct to raise hips as to use the bedpan q1h. 5. Heelbos. Remove q shift for 1 hour. 6. Wound inspection if no dressing q shift.

SUMMARY

The expertise nurses possess in the nursing process directly influences their nursing excellence. The more varied and creative their assessment skills, the more varied and creative their nursing interventions. One never becomes a complete expert on the nursing process. With each new learning acquisition, another new and exciting dimension of care surfaces. It is through these continually changing dimensions that nurses can transcend the eight-hour job, making it into an eight-hour experience.

NOTES

1. Lynda Juall Carpenito, *Nursing Diagnosis/Application in Clinical Practice* (Philadelphia: J.B. Lippincott, 1983), 29.

2. D. Little and D. Carnevali, *Nursing Care Planning* (Philadelphia: J.B. Lippincott, 1969), 54–57.

3. Jean Watson, *Nursing: The Philosophy and Science of Caring* (Boston: Little, Brown, 1979), 17.

4. E.L. Rothweiler et al., *The Art and Science of Nursing* (Philadelphia: F.A. Davis, 1959), 479.

5. Ibid., 51.

6. Carpenito, 27–28.

7. Patricia Benner and Judith Wrubel, "Skilled Clinical Knowledge: The Value of Perceptual Awareness," *Journal of Nursing Administration* 12 (May 1982):11–14.

8. Carpenito, 15–18.

9. Carpenito, 27–29.

SUGGESTED READINGS

Aspinall, Mary Jo, and Christine Tanner. *Decision Making for Patient Care—Applying the Nursing Process*. New York: Appleton-Century-Crofts, 1981.

Carnevali, Doris. *Nursing Care Planning*, 3d ed. Philadelphia: J.B. Lippincott, 1983.

Carnevali, Doris, et al. *Diagnostic Reasoning in Nursing*. Philadelphia: J.B. Lippincott, 1984.

Carpenito, Lynda Juall. *Nursing Diagnosis: Application to Clinical Practice*. Philadelphia: J.B. Lippincott, 1983.

Coletta, Suzanne Smith. "Values Clarification in Nursing." *American Journal of Nursing* 78 (December 1978):2057.

Dossey, Barbara. "Perfecting Your Skill for Systematic Patient Assessment." *Nursing* 79 (February 1979):42–45.

Gordon, Marjorie. *Nursing Diagnosis Process and Application*. New York: McGraw-Hill, 1982.

Henderson, B. "Nursing Diagnosis: Theory and Practice." *Advanced Nursing Science* 1 (October 1978):75–83.

Kim, M., and D. Moritz (eds.). *Classification of Nursing Dx—Proceedings of the 3rd and 4th National Conferences*. New York: McGraw-Hill, 1981.

Kim, Mi Ja, et al. *Classification of Nursing Diagnoses—Proceedings of the 5th National Conference*. St. Louis: C.V. Mosby, 1984.

Porter, A., et al. "Patient Needs on Admission." *American Journal of Nursing* 77 (January 1977):112–113.

Symposium on Nursing Diagnoses. Nursing Clinics of North America, September 1979.

Uustal, D. "Values Clarification in Nursing: Application to Practice." *American Journal of Nursing* 78 (December 1978):2058–2063.

Nursing Diagnosis is a quarterly newsletter published by the National Group for Classification of Nursing Diagnosis. A subscription may be obtained by contacting:

North American Nursing Diagnosis Association
St. Louis University Department of Nursing
3525 Carolin Street
St. Louis, MO 63104
Cost: $5.00

Appendix 7–A

Guidelines for Preparing Diagnostic Categories

A. The diagnostic category has three parts:
   1. The category label
   2. Etiological subcategory
   3. Defining characteristics
B. The criteria for each part are
   1. The category label
      a. Clear and concise (two or three words)
      b. Specific enough to be clinically useful
      c. Represents a clinical entity that a nurse can identify and treat
   2. Etiological subcategory (if it can be identified)
      a. Describes one probable cause of the health problem
      b. Directs interventions when combined with label
      c. Clear and concise, but specificity is vital
   3. Defining characteristics
      a. Observable signs and symptoms that are present
      b. Differentiation between critical defining characteristics and others
C. Independent nurse rating
   Rate the diagnostic category as to the degree of independent nursing interventions commonly involved in preventing, treating, or resolving the health problem using the following rating terms: High, Medium, Low.
D. Supporting literature
   Literature to support category label, etiological subcategory and/or defining characteristics (if available)
   National Group for Classification of Nursing Diagnosis
E. Suggested format
   1. Category label
   2. Etiological factors
   3. Defining characteristics (asterisk the critical one(s))

4. Degree of independent nursing therapy
   High   Medium   Low   (Circle one.)
5. Supportive literature

Source: National Group for Classification of Nursing Diagnosis, St. Louis University Department of Nursing, St. Louis, Missouri 63104.

Chapter 8

Communication and Clinical Instruction

Therapeutic communication is the core of successful professional nursing. Daily interactions with clients, their families, and members of the health team make the art of communication vital for professional nurses. Communication is the foundation upon which the nursing process is based and the basis for all effective nurse-client interactions. Therapeutic communication is the single most important skill a professional nurse can apply to attain professional autonomy (see Exhibit 8–1).

The nurse must value the effect of good therapeutic communications on the well-being of the client in order to incorporate this activity into all aspects of client care. This internalization of the concept provides a framework for the achievement of all levels of the hierarchy for autonomy in nursing.

Communicating effectively with others should be of prime concern to all professional nurses. Unfortunately, many practicing nurses fail to develop effective communication skills. They may be hampered by numerous factors; however, often the inability to communicate effectively may be attributed to certain myths that have been accepted as characteristics of "professional" nurses. These are that (1) "professionals" must solve the client's problems and (2) that "professionals" are always in control of their own emotions. Nurses who subscribe to these beliefs will develop a communication style that is aimed at solving client's problems while permitting them to maintain their emotional composure.

The first myth, that nurses can solve the client's problems, creates frustration and anxiety for nurses when they find that they cannot be successful. As professionals, nurses interact with clients in order that feelings and concerns can be shared and discussed. Nurses strive to "make everything better" but find that instead they are limited in their abilities to solve other people's problems. Nurses must accept the fact that fear, loss, and death are real concerns and cannot be eliminated by nursing efforts. Individuals who are suffering (physically and emotionally) can be best aided by a nonjudgmental listener who encourages them

167

Exhibit 8–1 Hierarchy for Autonomy in Nursing

to express their feelings and conveys that it is alright to have such emotions. This behavior will demonstrate sincerity and warmth to the client.

Nurses are often described as cold, insensitive, and uncaring individuals. Although this is not true of most nurses, such an outward appearance may be indicative of the second myth, that professionals are always in control of their emotions. To many, being in control of emotions is synonymous with efficient and effective nursing. Thus, displaying of emotions connotes an ineffective, non-professional failure.

In order to effectively communicate, nurses must first acknowledge and accept their own personal vulnerability. As human beings, nurses have emotions of sadness, fear, and frustration. To deny the existence of these feelings is to deny one's own humanity. Nurses have a responsibility to encourage individuals to share, to indicate that they accept the client's responses to the situation, and to convey that they are emotionally involved. This emotional involvement is often quite difficult for nurses to incorporate into their nursing practice. However, pride and personal satisfaction soon replace all personal discomfort as nurses realize they have made a positive difference in the life of a client.

Nurses who communicate superficially practice a technique called *emotional distancing*. Emotional distancing occurs in a situation when the professional nurse does not enter into the relationship at an affective level. Instead of establishing an interaction that relates feelings and emotions, communication is kept at a conversational, interviewing, or information-giving level. These nurses will consciously or unconsciously avoid topics and conversations that make them emotionally uncomfortable and vulnerable. Characteristics that identify emotional distancing include:

1. Use of cliches, e.g., "Don't worry, it will turn out fine." "Everything will turn out for the best."

2. Failure to display sadness to clients and families, e.g., through touch, tears, or words of comfort
3. Preoccupation with technical aspects of care, e.g., making frequent visits to check the IV
4. Avoidance of clients who are emotionally threatening, e.g., the terminally ill client

It is important that nurses and students disregard these myths and practice effective communication skills based on sound interpersonal relationships. The ability to communicate effectively is not automatic, however. It is a planned and learned skill involving practice and caring in order to be successful.

LEVELS OF COMMUNICATION

Five levels of communication are relevant to professional nursing:

1. *Conversational.* The conversational level of communication deals with causal and impersonal information. It involves issues of relatively little importance to either of the individuals participating in the interaction. A discussion of the weather or a football game would fall in this category.
2. *Interviewing.* The purpose of interviewing is to obtain information from an individual on a factual basis. Usually, there is very little emotional involvement in the topic and material being discussed. Filling out a form for admission to the health agency would be an example of this type of communication. The nursing history interview, however, incorporates interviewing the counseling for data collection.
3. *Information giving.* The third level of communication includes a wide range of communication interactions. It may be a brief encounter, with the client receiving information about where to go for physical therapy, or it can involve an intensive educational program on nutrition, exercises, or wellness. There may be some emotional involvement in this level if the shared material is related to the health and well-being of the client.
4. *Counseling.* Communication at the counseling level is the most important and hardest for the health professional because it deals with feelings and emotions. Counseling is the sharing of concerns, problems, and feelings and involves active listening on the part of the participants. It seeks as its goal the development of self-awareness and understanding, the fulfillment of personal needs, and the reduction of frustrations and anxieties.
5. *Psychotherapy.* Psychotherapy is a specified therapeutic technique used while caring for clients with mental health problems. It promotes behavioral change and involves counseling in much more depth and by specially

prepared individuals. It deals with the severe anxieties of individuals who exhibit changes in their mental health and patterns of behavior. This level is used only by the professional nurse who has had additional and more intense education in the techniques of clinical psychology.

Most nurse-client interactions occur on the first four levels; the fifth level requires special training and education. The first two levels present few problems because they deal with facts that are readily offered. The third level, information giving, involves preparation by the professional nurse to convey appropriate information to the client while utilizing all the principles of learning and teaching. Skill in health education should be a priority in the nursing practice of the professional nurse and can be developed through training and practice. The fourth level is crucial and, excluding psychotherapy, the most difficult in which to develop proficiency.

COMMUNICATION SKILLS

Communication can be identified as a major thread in the conceptual framework of most professional nursing curricula. Emphasis on communication techniques can be incorporated into the clinical focus of any nursing course. The learning objectives presented in Exhibit 8–2 related to one-to-one interactions could be considered as a separate focus or as the goal of part of another clinical experience.

Teaching the principles of therapeutic communication and promoting competency in exercising communication skills is a major task for the nurse educator, who must be knowledgeable and competent in these skills as well as able to encourage student learning in these areas. The nurse educator must be able to serve as a model of the objectives listed in Exhibit 8–2.

Exhibit 8–2 One-to-One Interactions

LEARNING OBJECTIVES: At the completion of the semester, the student will

1. Demonstrate caring and sincerity in communications
2. Utilize appropriate nonverbal techniques to promote mutual nurse-client interactions
3. Utilize appropriate verbal techniques to promote mutual nurse-client interactions
4. Avoid conversational habits that hinder effective nurse-client interactions and enhance emotional distancing

Caring and Sincerity in Communications

Nursing is the art of caring and the science of care giving. Nursing personnel must care in order to be effective care givers. Caring can be identified in nurses who demonstrate kindness, compassion, and empathy in their nurse-client interactions.

Sincerity is essential to the communication process as the nurse develops trusting relationships with clients. It is the foundation for all therapeutic communications and the basis for quality professional nursing care. Sincerity cannot be a learned skill; it is an inherent quality that is attitudinal.

Acceptance is a quality that is very important to the communication process. It is based on the idea that the communicators have infinite worth and dignity. The professional nurse establishes a trusting relationship during the nurse-client interaction by supporting the client during the communication. Low esteem can hinder a sharing of ideas and concerns by the client. Only by promoting the client's individual and unquestionable importance to the interaction can the professional nurse establish a bond of openness and sharing.

To teach and foster sincerity, caring, and acceptance in students, the nurse educator must function as a role model. Most learning that occurs originates from what the teacher does, not what the teacher says. The nursing instructor who advocates empathetic health care must display sincere empathy in teaching students and caring for clients. Specific teaching strategies are presented at the end of this chapter.

Nonverbal Techniques To Promote Mutual Nurse-Client Interactions

In a culture that values quick responses, the use of nonverbal communication techniques in nurse-client interactions is of paramount importance. Active listening, silence, touch, and body language are nonverbal components of most nurse-client interactions.

Active Listening

People who do not voluntarily expend more than half their energies listening to the communications of others are not actively listening. Active listening is not a passive process, for it requires great concentration and effort on the part of the listener. Few people listen objectively and actively to the communication of others; instead, they dwell on their own thoughts and develop other blocks to listening. Active listeners provide their partners in communication the opportunity to share thoughts and concerns with an interested and empathetic individual.

The elements of active listening include:

- channeling attention to the sender and staying quiet within oneself
- reducing or eliminating barriers
- maintaining eye contact
- "squaring off" eye to eye, shoulder to shoulder
- avoiding interruptions

Barriers to active listening are always present, and the professional nurse must take the appropriate measures of eliminating them or their influence on an interaction. Students should be aware of the following possible blocks to active listening:

1. Internal

   - The person's views are different from the nurse's perceptions.
   - The person's dialect or accent is different.
   - The person's appearance is different or distracting.
   - The person is in pain or is anxious.
   - The person is telling the nurse something that he or she does not want to hear.
   - The nurse feels a dislike toward the person.
   - The nurse is thinking of something else.
   - The nurse is planning the next statement.
   - The nurse is anxious or apprehensive.

2. External

   - noise from equipment, speakers, television, radios, etc.
   - lack of privacy
   - physical hinderances such as desks, equipment, space, etc.
   - verbal remarks such as clichés, trite comments, or interruptions

After learning the principles of active listening, students should be assigned to participate as active listeners in a dialogue with a fellow student (see Exhibit 8–3). The goal of this exercise is to demonstrate the effectiveness of active listening and its use in all personal interactions. Barriers to productive interaction can be dealt with during the communication process, and students will have the opportunity to relate their feelings and concerns immediately after the experience.

Exhibit 8–3 An Exercise in Active Listening

(Choose a student partner.)

1. Partner 1 tells partner 2 about the death of a person or animal remembered most vividly and why the memory is so vivid. (Time limit: 10 minutes)
2. Partner 2 practices active listening, utilizing the principles of eye contact, body language, silence, and touch.
3. Switch roles.
4. Discuss.

Answer the following:

1. When you were the speaker what kind of verbal and nonverbal messages did the listener send you?
2. What is your reaction to active listening for ten minutes? What did you learn?
3. Are you usually an active listener?

Silence

Second only to active listening in importance as a nonverbal therapeutic communication technique is the use of silence. In nursing this can be defined as the period of time during which the nurse waits without interrupting the client's thought process. Such a silence can occur while waiting for the client to speak or allowing the client time to collect his or her thoughts. With silence, there is always some time for nonverbal interaction. Silence provides the time for

- the communicators to assess each other
- each to organize thoughts and plan for the next verbal exchange
- the client and nurse to sit quietly, accepting and trusting each other
- a quietness that promotes calm in the face of anger
- conveying feelings and emotions to each other when words are not enough

Most people feel uncomfortable with silence and continually attempt to cover silence with a verbal exchange. During dialogue with individual students, the nurse educator can assess the learner's interpretation of silence and feelings about it. Students can be directed to identify their comfort or lack of comfort by using silence in a group. Students who find themselves uncomfortable with silence can incorporate the communication technique into interactions by interjecting five- to ten-second periods of silence. Gradually they should discover they no longer feel the need to fill every silence with conversation. Silence can be a very effective communication technique to show caring. The death of a client to whom you have felt close may evoke such sorrow that the only consolation you can offer the client's family is to say "I don't know what to say," and then be silent.

Touch

The third nonverbal communication technique is touch. Touching always communicates something to a coparticipant in an interaction. The recipient's interpretation of this nonverbal technique will depend upon what meaning the recipient attaches to the action. The need to touch is universal; the amount is individual. Touch can be an effective tool in conveying concern and deep emotion. It can show support and empathy for what the client is saying as well as feeling.

Touch is often hindered in the clinical setting by physical, emotional, and aesthetic barriers. Equipment in a client's room such as tubing, isolation screens, wheelchairs, pumps, croupettes, and so on are physical barriers that may inhibit the use of touch as an essential form of communication. Emotional barriers such as psychological stress, fear, misinterpretation, and mistrust may also prevent the nonverbal interaction of touching. Aesthetic barriers to communication by touch include physical deformities, strong odors, and lesions.

The creative educator can promote touching as a communication tool by engaging in its use when appropriate and encouraging students to do so in their nursing care. Leaving a critically ill client's hand uncovered should encourage touch amidst all the intensive care equipment. Families should be encouraged to touch loved ones who are under care, even during hours of silent communication.

Parents must also be reassured that it is all right for them to touch their hospitalized child. Medical procedures and equipment should not prevent parents from holding their child and sharing their love by touch. If there are periods of time when the parents cannot be with the child, a special effort should be made to provide them with time to hold, touch, and love the child. Providing parents with an opportunity to bathe their child can be very therapeutic for both the child and the parents. The professional nurse should use touch as a key assessment factor in evaluating parent-child bonding. Without the knowledge that touch is important to the child in the hospital, parents might keep their distance, giving a false impression of their relationship with their child. It is therefore very important that all parents and families be encouraged to use touch as nonverbal communication when interacting with the individual receiving care in a health agency.

The student nurse can be guided to use touch as a nonverbal therapeutic communication tool by the creative nurse educator, learning to use touch routinely and naturally in providing quality health care. Thus it is important that students be able to observe and evaluate the use of touch in the clinical setting and its application to nursing practice.

Students can assess the presence of touch, or lack of it, with the exercises in Exhibit 8–4. These activities can be incorporated into one clinical focus sheet or used separately whenever appropriate.

Exhibit 8–4 Exercises Related to Touching

1. Identify the factors in the client's environment that would promote or deter the use of touch.
2. Identify factors related to the client or the client's family that would promote or deter the use of touch.
3. Assess the client's response to touch as a therapeutic communication tool.
4. List the nursing interventions that would encourage the use of touch in caring for the client.

Body Language

The use of body language as a technique of therapeutic communication can be applied to all nurse-client interactions. Body language includes posture and eye contact. During therapeutic interactions, the nurse and the client should communicate at the same physical level. The communicators should sit or stand facing each other so that their shoulders form an invisible square. This alignment reduces external distraction while promoting active listening.

Keeping the shoulders at an even level also enhances the nurse-client interaction because it prevents feelings of inferiority created when one stands over another. Hospitalized clients are often placed in dependent positions that do nothing to facilitate independent decision making on the part of the client. A knowledgeable nurse can circumvent this by thoughtful positioning of the client or the nurse to promote independence. Clients should be placed in a sitting position whenever possible so that they can feel "up." Sitting up will enable them to assert themselves more easily and make appropriate decisions about their health care.

Nurse educators should apply the principle of shoulder-to-shoulder communication in teacher-student interactions. This promotes self-esteem in the student communicator and places the communicators on an equal footing. It suggests that the educator is really listening and cares about what the student is saying. By using body posture in teacher-student interactions, the educator will subtly promote the use of this technique by the student in nurse-client communications.

Eye Contact

The literature concerning eye contact or the lack of it is voluminous. In regard to therapeutic communication, two types of eye contact should be considered: (1) habitually poor eye contact and (2) eye contact that changes abruptly during an interaction. The person with habitual lack of eye contact creates discomfort in a partner to a dialogue. The caring person should express the discomfort, naming its source, in an effort to improve future interactions with the person whose eye contact is poor. It is not necessary to uncover the reasons for lack of eye contact, but only to discuss its presence and methods of rectifying the problem. With conscious effort a person can learn to communicate while maintaining direct eye contact.

Abrupt change in a client's eye contact during an interaction should also be queried in a very honest but caring manner. It is usually beneficial to inquire as to the meaning of a break in eye contact. The reason for the change may be related to the topic of communication or may be an internal stress such as pain. If the nurse acknowledges the change in nonverbal communication, the client may be helped to deal with a previously unexpressed problem or concern.

The nurse educator must deal with the students in teacher-student interactions in the same manner. Students with poor eye contact must be dealt with individually in an effort to increase their communication skills. Students who realize they have a problem maintaining eye contact can begin to take appropriate steps to correct this nonverbal barrier to communication. This will enhance all interactions of the student whether personal or professional.

Verbal Techniques To Promote Mutual Nurse-Client Interactions

Communication techniques signified by the term *therapeutic* are often viewed by students as artificial or forced and unnatural. A conflict emerges in students who think that if they practice therapeutic communication with clients, they cannot be themselves. They think of therapeutic communication as playing a role, with the techniques reserved for client interactions only. Many students also believe that by using therapeutic communication techniques, they will force the client to reveal details and problems that normally should not be discussed. Using these skills for purposes of client manipulation is a valid concern and something that should be avoided at all times. During the educational process, the nurse instructor should stress the proper use of these techniques and should discourage using them to pry into the client's private thoughts and feelings.

Students frequently believe that they have only two alternatives:

1. To use therapeutic communication techniques for all clients and practice their own communication style in all other interactions.
2. To reject therapeutic communication techniques altogether and use their own communication style in all interactions.

But a third alternative exists—that students each establish their own philosophy of communication, with an eclectic approach to all nurse-client techniques in order to develop their own styles. The style of communication chosen should be comfortable for the individual and prove effective in both private and professional interactions. The level of competency in communicating will directly influence the professional nurse's degree of nursing excellence. As with the learning of any skill, preparation and practice are essential. The verbal techniques that the professional nurse can use to promote high-quality health care are questioning, making observations, restating, reflecting, and encouraging solution finding.

Questioning

Through questioning, the professional nurse has the opportunity to assess the client's verbal and nonverbal responses. The client shares answers to the questions while developing a trusting relationship with the nurse. Through open-ended questions the professional nurse can convey that what the client is saying, feeling, and meaning matters. Open-ended questions begin with the words *who, what, when, where,* or *how* and require the client to provide explanations. Asking the client "What do you mean by sharp pain?" encourages a detailed response that will provide the nurse with more information about the situation.

Closed-ended questions not only limit the client's responses but convey very little caring or empathy from the professional nurse to the client. Closed-ended questions—such as "Do you have pain?"—require only one-word or two-word answers and do not encourage the client to share feelings and concerns. Professional nurses should be careful to avoid using this type of questioning to collect data for a nursing history. If closed-ended questions are used, they will receive only the responses required by the assessment form, not incidental assessment data vital for the development of a nursing care plan.

Observations

Making observations about what the client has said or has not said is a very important therapeutic communications technique. The professional nurse uses this communication skill to assess the verbal and nonverbal responses of the client and share this information with the client. An interaction using this technique might sound like this:

> *Nurse:* How are you feeling?
> *Client:* Fine, I guess. [Intonation suggests that all is *not* fine.]
> *Nurse:* You say you guess you are fine, but your voice sounds as if all is not fine.

Making observations about the client's speech patterns, body posture, eye contact, and other important nonverbal communication is an important part of therapeutic communications. It affords the client the opportunity to review what was said as compared with what was really meant. It also clarifies the statements of the client in case the nurse has misinterpreted the client's communication.

Reflection

The hardest communication technique for the professional to use effectively is related to reflection. It is used to convey to the client the nurse's understanding of what has just been said. Effective reflection requires quick thinking, for the response to the client should be immediate. Reflection can be defined as the repeating of the client's words as the nurse hears them, the client's meaning as interpreted by the nurse, or the client's nonverbal communication as perceived by the nurse. This method of therapeutic communication is used to help clients explore their own reasoning and clarify what has been said. An example of each follows:

Reflection of words
Complete
Client: I get very angry when the doctor will not listen to me.
Nurse: You get very angry when the doctor will not listen to you?

Partial
Client: I can't stop crying. I know my husband cannot be here every day.
Nurse: You are so homesick.

Reflection of meaning
Client: I don't want to have this test done. [Crying]
Nurse: You are afraid to have the test done because of what it might show.

Reflection of nonverbal communication
Client: [Client is crying.] I am all right.
Nurse: This must be very upsetting for you.

Using reflection as a therapeutic tool of communication can be very crucial to the success of the nurse-client relationship. It is important, however, for the professional nurse to know when to use this technique and to recognize the pitfalls of its habitual use. For effective results the professional nurse must judiciously decide with whom to use the technique of reflection and how much is appropriate. Constant reflection *can* sound artificial or convey disinterest and passive listening to the client. Reflection must be coupled with sensitivity if it is to be used effectively and must be used only in an atmosphere of sincere warmth and caring.

Summarizing

Of utmost importance to the nurse-client interaction is the summary or brief review of what communication has taken place. It provides both the client and the nurse a chance to evaluate the accuracy of information exchanged. Any misinformation can be identified at this time and the client can clarify portions of the interaction or ask pertinent questions of the nurse.

Avoiding Conversational Habits

Just as it is valuable for the professional nurse to know which types of verbal communication are appropriate and can enhance a nurse-client interaction, it is likewise important to understand what conversational habits can hinder communication. Some that can block therapeutic communication are using reassuring clichés, expressing approval or disapproval, advising, and changing the subject. The professional nurse should avoid the use of these types of exchanges because of their adverse effect on the client-nurse interaction.

Many times a nurse uses reassuring clichés in the sincere attempt to reduce a client's anxiety. Because clichés are part of the everyday conversation of most individuals, they provide time fillers when one does not know what to say or when the appropriate words are not readily available. Since they are so automatic, however, they are one of the most common communication blocks and nurses must make a special effort to eliminate them from their professional communication. The use of these trite remarks conveys to the client that the nurse feels the client is being silly, worrying needlessly, or that his or her concerns are unimportant. Responses such as "Everything will be all right," "Don't worry, everything will turn out for the best," or "Things could be a lot worse; you could have cancer," tell the client that the nurse does not understand what the client is feeling and does not really care.

Wishing to encourage or discourage a behavior in the client may signal an I-know-what-is-best-for-you attitude on the part of the nurse. Attempting to motivate the client to embrace the nurse's own values hinders expression of the client's own feelings and attitudes. Communication becomes blocked because the nurse is implying that there is a right and a wrong way to believe or feel about the concern and the nurse knows the right way. This prevents the client from speaking freely and exploring his or her feelings about the topic. Effective communication relies upon acceptance, but use of this type of conversational tool conveys acceptance only when the client agrees with the beliefs of the nurse. An example:

Wrong
Client: I know I shouldn't let this thing get to me.
Nurse: You are right. You must be strong.

Right
Nurse: This must be very difficult for you.
Client: It certainly is. I just feel as though . . .

Contradictions or implied disapproval may relay feelings of nonacceptance to which the client may react with silence in defense. It is vital that the professional nurse provide the client with the opportunity to express all thoughts and feelings without worrying about acceptance and judgment from health professionals.

Just as health professionals tend to make decisions and judgments for the client, they also function under the misconception that their advice is vitally important to the well-being and welfare of the client. A communication block occurs when the professional nurse tries to help by directing the client's life. Although this paternal attitude is inherent to the health professions, the professional nurse should assist clients in exploring their own feelings and ideas about topics of concern in order to arrive at their own solutions. If a client asks for a nurse's advice, it is best for the professional to reflect the question back to the client for further evaluation. Contrary to popular belief, the professional nurse does not always know what is best for the client and the client's family.

One of the easiest blocks to communication is changing the subject. In the nurse-client interaction it occurs for various reasons—from incorrect reflection of the client's feelings to a genuine attempt on the part of the nurse to ease the tension in the interaction. Another reason that the subject is changed by the professional is that, not knowing what else to say, the nurse may grasp at anything. The nurse must be constantly alert to this communication block and if it occurs should make every attempt to direct the interaction back to important aspects of the communication. Examples of this block are

Client: I am so worried about my four children.
Nurse: You have four children?

Client: I am so worried about my children.
Nurse: How many children do you have?

Client: I am so worried about my children. [Crying]
Nurse: Crying will make you feel better. [Handing her a tissue]

These examples show how the nurse failed to communicate effectively with the client about her concern for her children. An appropriate response to this statement might be "You are very worried about your children" or "It must be very hard for you to be here away from your children." Either would provide the client the opportunity to respond directly about her concerns for her children and keep the communication viable.

Internalizing Therapeutic Communication Techniques

Therapeutic techniques and blocks of communication have been presented here in the belief that it is important for all professional nurses to have a basic understanding of the tools of effective communication. It is also important that once learned, these tools of communication should become an integral part of the professional nurse's practice. Concentration on specific techniques should be avoided and emphasis should be placed instead upon the professional's attitude of caring, empathy, and compassion. Each nurse should be encouraged to be natural and incorporate individual personality and communication style into all nurse-client interactions. Professional nurses who keep this thought in mind while learning therapeutic communications techniques will function more effectively while still conveying the warmth and kindness that is so vital to the communications process.

Nurses often receive tacit messages that to be a professional one cannot be human. In a quest to deny their own human vulnerability, they build walls around the human self. To separate humanism from professionalism does not produce a more professional nurse, only a less caring human being. The clichés that nurses develop, such as "Don't worry," "Everything will be all right," or "Ask your doctor," satisfactorily cement their world from client penetration. The problem in professional nursing is not that one becomes too emotionally involved with the client, but that one *does not.*

TEACHING THERAPEUTIC COMMUNICATIONS

Teaching the principles of interpersonal communications and promoting effective communications in nursing students is a major task for nurse educators. Not only must they excel as instructors of nursing but they must also demonstrate expertise in the use of effective interpersonal communications. Since students learn more from what instructors do than from what they say, it is vital that nurse educators function as good role models. As effective communicators, nurse educators must display an attitude of caring, understanding, acceptance, and sincerity in their personal and professional interactions. These characteristics are essential components of the communication process, and their presence or absence in nurse educators will influence the learning process of students and all educator-student interactions.

Students enter the educational system with certain social skills related to communications. At birth, infants communicate to fulfill their basic needs, and as they grow and develop, children use communication as a mechanism for socialization and learning. These life experiences provide all persons with an extensive background in the area of interpersonal interactions. Thus, students admitted to nursing programs enter the educational setting with certain established patterns of communication. This incoming behavior should be recognized for its worth and be utilized in the development and refinement of goal-directed communications.

Nurse educators need to encourage students to use their own style of communication when interacting with clients. Instead of "unlearning" the previously acquired communications skills, students should be urged to capitalize upon all their knowledge and experience. Teaching to the weaknesses of students has been found to be ineffectual and a waste of time. Evaluations that constantly identify errors in the communications skills during client-nurse interactions are negative reinforcement and compel students to change their previously established communication patterns. This type of teaching convinces students that there is only one way to communicate effectively and that a misplaced "Uh, huh!" or "That's too bad!" will devastate the client and block any further communications.

The students' natural communication style should be supported and encouraged. Nurse educators must stress that there is no one "right" question to ask or response to be given. It is only when educators focus their attention on the strengths of these students' communication abilities that learning of effective communication skills can begin to occur. Maximizing students' assets will promote learning, application, and internalization of the techniques of effective interpersonal communications.

CREATIVE CLINICAL INSTRUCTION

Because teaching in the classroom lends itself to traditional methods of instruction, such as lecture, educators will often utilize these strategies in order to expedite preparation and in-class time. However, teaching of communications must provide nursing students with opportunities for exploration, experimentation, and feedback. Traditional methods of teaching therapeutic communications do not always provide these opportunities. Of course, nurse educators should not use a teaching strategy just because it is creative. They should evaluate both traditional and creative methods of teaching communications according to their effectiveness in promoting the transfer of communication theory to the clinical setting.

Process Recording

The use of process recordings to increase learning related to interpersonal communications is a very effective teaching strategy. Following a client-nurse interaction, students are to select a portion of the interaction (approximately five minutes) and write down the entire conversation. Seeing the actual words spoken provides an opportunity for students to evaluate the communication techniques that they utilized during the client-nurse interaction. The disadvantage of this teaching method is that it requires students to remember exactly what was said during the communication with the client. The content of the interaction must be written down verbatim in order for students to evaluate the effectiveness of their communication skills. Tape recording these interactions eliminates the need for students to remember the content, but it also tends to stifle a spontaneous exchange between the student and the client. Requiring a written evaluation of the effectiveness of the client-nurse interaction forces students to take an in-depth look at their communication skills and to better identify the strengths and weaknesses of their interpersonal communications. Exhibits 8–5 and 8–6 indicate how the procedure would work.

Role Play

Role play is a type of simulation that provides the student with insight into real-life situations. The educator should select situations that would be applicable to

---

Exhibit 8–5 Guidelines for Process Recordings

> 1. Develop an appropriate relationship with a selected client.
> 2. Select an excerpt from your communication with the client and write the interaction on the Nurse-Client Interaction Sheet. This must be written verbatim.
> *3. On the Nurse-Client Interaction Sheet, complete the following:
>   A. Identify factors that assisted in establishing the relationship.
>   B. Identify factors that hindered the relationship.
>   C. Summarize your evaluation of the interaction with the client as to its effectiveness.
> *See Nurse/Client Interaction Sheet.

Exhibit 8–6 Nurse-Client Interaction Sheet

Nurse Communication	*Client Communication*	*Evaluation*
A.		
B.		
C.		

students' present learning needs. For example, if students are working in pediatrics, a situation involving a distraught mother would be appropriate. A student portraying the mother is provided with enough information to develop the role. Another student, representing the nurse, is given the same information and instructed to use appropriate communication skills in dealing with the upset parent. This interaction will usually take only five minutes before maximum learning has occurred. If the interchange continues beyond this point, it becomes repetitious and productivity will be lost.

The educator can also select clinical situations for role play that are emotionally difficult for students. For example, the instructor could develop a situation that deals with a client being told a new diagnosis of a terminal illness, a client who is dying, or a family of a child who is having major life-threatening surgery. The actual role play would occur in the same manner as the previously described one relating to the distraught mother. However, this situation would focus on the emotional aspects of the nurse dealing with "difficult" interactions.

The nurse educator can ask students what questions they are most afraid a client will ask in emotionally charged interchanges. These questions can be incorporated into the role play and discussed by the class at the end of the interaction. Because fear of certain questions may keep students away from the client and family both physically and mentally, the point should be emphasized that there is no one best answer to these inquiries. Students need to learn that it is alright to say "I don't have the answers to why this has happened," "I feel sad that this is happening. Is there any way I can help you?" or "I don't know what to say!" The instructor must stress that it is alright to cry with clients and families and to do so shows strength in professionalism, not weakness or lack of control. At this time, emotional distancing can be discussed and the barriers that it creates when dealing with clients and their families.

After the role play, the nurse educator asks the participants for their evaluation. The educator should encourage the students to identify areas where the conversation was blocked and areas where participants responded appropriately. The entire class can then offer criticisms about the communication, which helps all the students in future interactions. This activity is a learning experience, and the educator should not permit the class to ridicule and belittle the participants. Instead students should be encouraged to contribute suggestions for ways of improving the interpersonal communications.

Audiovisuals

The nurse educator should consider the use of audiovisuals when teaching interpersonal communications. This strategy can be used in two major ways. Tape recording an interview between the instructor and another person can be used to convey the proper method of communicating with others. The students can listen to the audiotapes of this interaction and identify the appropriate response to client questions and concerns. Since a great deal of communication is through nonverbal cues, the lack of visual content may limit student learning.

The videotape can be used in the same manner as the audiotape with the advantage of visual content. Unlike dramatization, the interaction on videotape can be a spontaneous exchange between the educator and another individual. This spontaneity promotes a more "natural" interaction for the demonstration of effective interpersonal communication skills. After the videotape has been completed, it can then be evaluated by the nurse educator for content and appropriate study guides can be developed for use by the students. This method of teaching interpersonal communications eliminates the need for the time-consuming task of writing a script, yet provides the student with a similar simulation experience.

Another use of audiovisuals is for students to record their own interactions on audiotape and then critically evaluate the results. This provides an excellent mechanism for students to receive feedback about their interactions. By hearing or seeing themselves in real situations, students can honestly and accurately evaluate the effectiveness of the interaction and the achievement of designated goals. The audiotape lends itself more readily to this teaching strategy than the videotape because the equipment is more available to students and educators; and the size of the equipment encourages its use outside the classroom.

Videotaping student interactions is more difficult than audiotaping exchanges because equipment for the former is bigger, costlier, and less mobile. Although its use is generally limited to a studio, portable equipment may be available for use outside the educational facility. If so, this educational tool can be taken to the client to film client-nurse interactions. Videotaping in a natural setting provides students with an opportunity to evaluate their interpersonal communication skills more realistically.

If portable equipment is not accessible, videotaping can still be very beneficial. Students can videotape communications with other individuals in the studio or classroom. After viewing the tape, the students can readily identify strengths and weaknesses in their communications by seeing nonverbal cues as well as hearing the verbal exchange. The videotape also provides the educator with a means of evaluating the progress of the student in developing effective communication skills.

Role Modeling

Role modeling by the educator is a very effective means of teaching students the proper method of communications. The instructor interacts with a client and/or family while the student is present. Utilizing appropriate techniques of communication, the educator deals with the situation and helps the individuals with their concerns. The following is an example of role modeling.

> *Situation.* A 77-year-old female terminally ill with metastatic cancer can no longer swallow. The physician telephones an order for a nasogastric tube for feedings. The student caring for the client is very upset and expresses a concern that the family has not been informed or given any options. The instructor and student discuss the alternatives, but the student is reluctant to communicate these with the family because of his inexperience. The educator assumes the role of the professional nurse practitioner and the student becomes an observer. After the introductions, a dialogue between the educator and the patient's son might proceed in this manner:
>
> *Educator:* What is wrong with your mother?
> *Son:* She is dying.
> *Educator:* Yes, she is. Your mother can no longer eat and the physician wants a feeding tube inserted. How do you feel about this?
> *Son:* I don't know. I just don't want her to suffer.
> *Educator:* You don't want her to suffer.
> *Son:* She has been through so much already. Will the tube help her?
> *Educator:* It will probably prolong her life.
> *Son:* I don't know if that is such a good idea. Will the tube annoy her?
> *Educator:* Yes, usually. It is somewhat uncomfortable.
> *Son:* Oh.
> *Educator:* I would like to share with you some of the possible alternatives you have concerning this, and the choices available to you. You can consent to a feeding tube, refuse the feeding tube, refuse all treatments except comfort measures, or do everything possible to prolong life. Please keep in mind that, whatever decision you make, our nursing goal for your mother is making her as comfortable as possible.
> *Son:* I will have to think about it. But if she is going to die anyway, it seems to make sense to make her comfortable but not to prolong it.

After the role-modeling demonstration the student and the educator review what has been said. Any questions the student might have about the interaction should be answered and discussed at length if appropriate. The interaction can then be shared with the entire clinical group during post-conference and students' concerns and questions discussed. Often when students have an opportunity to witness the nurse educator interacting with clients, it reinforces the importance of utilizing good communication skills in practicing professional nursing.

Independent Study

Independent study can be used by students to learn the basics for developing effective interpersonal communications skills. Students can learn the communication process and specific communication skills through selected readings, audiovisual materials, and written assignments. However, the disadvantage of utilizing independent study as a major teaching tool for learning interpersonal communications is that the knowledge acquired must be supplemented by one or more of the teaching strategies that focus on practice.

Independent study can be used to promote the application of the principles of therapeutic communications. The most obvious method of learning the practical aspects of communication is for students to utilize these skills in their daily interactions. This does not mean that these techniques should be misused for manipulative purposes or to maneuver people to reveal feelings and concerns that they wish to keep private. Instead, students should be encouraged to practice their communication skills with family, friends, and other students who wish to assist in the learning process. If students use these techniques in all their communications, the skills will become an integral part of their lives, and the internalization of these principles will occur more easily.

SUMMARY

The ability to communicate is not intuitive. It is the result of many hard hours of learning, practicing, and internalizing. Because of its relationship to nursing, therapeutic communications must be presented as a vital part of professional practice. A nurse educator must internalize the importance of good communication techniques in order to convey to students their role in professional nursing. The principles of therapeutic communication must be put into practice with clients and students. It is essential that clinical instructors promote the integration of appropriate communication skills and techniques into the personal and professional lives of all individuals involved in the nursing profession.

SUGGESTED READINGS

Almore, Mary G. "Dyadic Communication." *American Journal of Nursing* 79 (June 1979):1076–1078.

Bartnick, Roger W., and Charles R. O'Brien. "Health Care and Counseling Skills." *The Personnel and Guidance Journal* 58 (June 1980):666–667.

Collins, Mattie. *Communication in Health Care.* St. Louis: C.V. Mosby, 1977.

Edwards, Barba, and John Brillhart. *Communication in Nursing Practice.* St. Louis: C.V. Mosby, 1981.

Hein, Eleanor. *Communication in Nursing Practice.* Boston: Little, Brown, 1980.

Karns, Phyllis J., and Therese A. Schwab. "Therapeutic Communication and Clinical Instruction." *Nursing Outlook* 30 (January 1982):39–43.

Jungman, Lynne B. "When Your Feelings Get in the Way." *American Journal of Nursing* 79 (June 1979):1074–1075.

Long, Lynetter, and Sister P. Prophit. *Understanding/Responding; A Communication Manual for Nurses*. Belmont, Calif.: Wadsworth, 1981.

Peplau, Hildegard E. *Interpersonal Relations in Nursing*. New York: G.P. Putnam, 1952.

Ramackers, Mary James. "Communication Blocks Revisited." *American Journal of Nursing* 79 (June 1979):1079–1081.

Smith, Voncile M., and Thelma A. Bass. *Communication for Health Professionals*. Philadelpha: J.B. Lippincott, 1979.

Waddell, Elizabeth. "Quality Touching to Communicate Caring." *Nursing Forum* 18 (1979):288–292.

Chapter 9

Assertiveness and Clinical Instruction

After a nurse has made a commitment to accountability, personal and professional, this commitment is made operational through deliberate, open collaborative behavior. Practicing nurses interact assertively, nonassertively, or aggressively, and each behavior influences their relationships. Collaboration is important, but is not initiated by the nonassertive nurse because of fear and is not accepted from the aggressive nurse because of hostility.

Nonassertiveness is behavior that demonstrates negative self-worth by allowing others to infringe on one's rights. At the other extreme is aggressive behavior, which is manipulative and domineering; the sole goal is getting one's way with tactics that infringe on the rights of others. Assertion is distinct from nonassertion and aggression, although it involves certain positive aspects of each of the other two styles of behavior. The assertive person demonstrates a belief in the importance of the fundamental rights of all human beings. This person states personal desires or goals honestly without infringing on the rights of others. The goal of assertive behavior is to make relationships better (see Exhibit 9–1).

Assertiveness is not a magical acquisition but must be learned just like any other valuable behavioral skill. Learners must apply belief in the basic human rights to themselves and support their own self-worth, self-esteem, and personal dignity. The process of learning assertiveness must be structured in such a way as to produce continued motivation. The end product will prove to be the most valued skill one could acquire, and will automatically enable the nurse to put into operation commitment to accountability and the nursing profession (see Exhibit 9–2).

People acquire a pattern of responding to stressors in their lives. Some patterns manage stress constructively while others are destructive. Interestingly, some individuals utilize constructive strategies in their professional life and destructive in their personal life or vice versa. Exhibit 9–3 illustrates examples of direct and indirect constructive or destructive strategies.

Exhibit 9–1 Nonassertive, Aggressive, and Assertive Behaviors

	Definition	*Characteristics*	*Appearance*
Nonassertive	allowing others to infringe on your rights by denying your own importance, inviting victimization	apologetic hesitant dishonest negative self-worth	fidgety poor eye contact stooped posture soft voice
Aggressive	stating your desires, goals, dislikes by intentionally infringing on the rights of others	dominating sarcastic flippant alienating hurtful	loud rigid posture clenched fists
Assertive	stating your desires, goals, dislikes humanistically while actively listening to the concerns of others	honest sincere caring respectful direct	firm, relaxed voice erect posture appropriate eye contact

Exhibit 9–2 The Assertiveness Spectrum

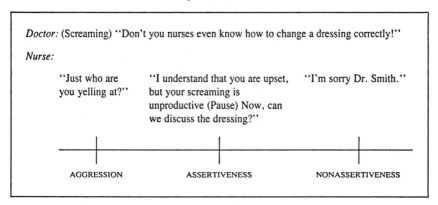

Doctor: (Screaming) "Don't you nurses even know how to change a dressing correctly!"

Nurse:

| "Just who are you yelling at?" | "I understand that you are upset, but your screaming is unproductive (Pause) Now, can we discuss the dressing?" | "I'm sorry Dr. Smith." |

AGGRESSION   ASSERTIVENESS   NONASSERTIVENESS

An assertive person responds honestly and empathetically, avoiding the guilt and frustration that accompany nonassertive passivity as well as the loss of control and the manipulation of overt and covert aggression. When you respond by saying "Yes" or nothing at all to a situation where you really wish to say "No," then you are requesting abuse, frustration, disrespect, and ultimately the illnesses associated with the stress that results. You are condoning others' irresponsible behavior and sanctioning further "put-downs" and personal violations. This, in turn, lowers self-esteem and makes you feel valueless professionally and personally. As a result, dishonest relationships are promoted and breakdowns in communication occur.

Exhibit 9–3 Patterns of Coping with Stress

	Constructive (active)	*Destructive* (passive)
Direct	• Changing the source of the stress • Confronting source • Adopting a positive attitude	• Ignoring the source of the stress • Avoiding the source • Leaving
Indirect	• Talking about the source of stress • Changing yourself • Getting involved in other activities (exercise, relaxation techniques)	• Alcohol, drugs, food, tobacco • Getting ill • Collapsing

Assertiveness cannot be discussed without including an explanation of risk taking and its applicability to clinical instruction. Risk taking is an activity that involves a varying degree of psychological or physical danger. In certain situations the danger entailed by assertive behavioral responses may range from very high (job loss) to very low (being ignored). Each individual assigns a degree of risk to each experience that involves assertion, nonassertion, or aggression on the basis of one's life experiences. The degree of risk perceived by the individual will influence behavioral patterns and responses. Thus, the degree of risk taking and its importance in all situations can only be determined by the person involved.

FEMALE BEHAVIORAL NORMS

The origins of nonassertive behavior of the nurse as a member of the health team are twofold. The majority of nurses are female, and according to the traditional sex norms established by our society and culture, females were supposed to be nonassertive. The female who enters the nursing profession has nonassertiveness reinforced by another set of norms, those dictating her role relative to other members of the health team. Historically, the nurse has been subordinate to all other members of the health team and especially submissive to physicians. The sociological etiology of female nonassertion is extensive. Much has been written on the subject (see the suggested readings at the end of this chapter).

The socialization of women begins in infancy. The responses adults make to certain behaviors of girls and boys encourage or discourage the behavior. Girls are encouraged to be dependent, quiet, gentle, and more sensitive to pain, while this same behavior is discouraged in boys. Unlike their female counterparts male children are conversely encouraged to be aggressive, inquisitive, and active.[1] As the female matures, she learns what behavior society expects when it rewards her passivity and dependency. For example, the teenage girl who is extremely competitive in the classroom and the girl who excels on the basketball court may not be busy with Saturday night dates. On the other hand, the "pretty blond" and the "nice girl" are very attractive as dates to the adolescent male.

To see how individuals have been sociologically conditioned into sex roles, consider a learning exercise from *The New Assertive Woman*.[2] Participants at an assertiveness training course were asked to list nouns and adjectives to describe female and male traits. The following are the most typical responses elicited:

Female Nonassertive	Male Nonassertive	Female Aggressive	Male Aggressive
Kind	Wishy-washy	Bitchy	Confident
Pleasant	Pansy	Pushy	Successful

This exercise demonstrates how people have been conditioned to accept or reject certain behaviors solely on gender.

EDUCATION VERSUS REALITY

Nursing before the nineteenth century was disorganized and unstructured. It was provided by religious orders who tended the spirit and other women "of questionable morals" who tended the body. In an attempt to improve nursing care, training schools were founded on the philosophy of the religious orders. Self-abnegation, dedication, and strict obedience to authority were the guiding principles.[3]

Nursing education has, by and large, moved away from its previously hospital-controlled schools into colleges and universities. Nurses ask themselves whether their guiding principles have changed or whether they continue to expect of their students nineteenth-century behavior. Herman describes the paradoxical messages with which students are confronted:

1. To be independent as far as nursing knowledge and practice go, but to retain such values as sacrifice and humility. Do not question or challenge issues that indicate your competence or knowledge.
2. To practice with a sound professional scientific knowledge base, but not to become emotionally involved with patients, co-workers or issues—maintain a professional role. Ignore conflict, deny your feelings and those of patients or co-workers—keep the environment calm and tension free.
3. To be professional, but not to expect equal professional financial reimbursement despite educational background and work performed.
4. To be an equal member of the health care team, but not to participate in policy-making or decisions. Never compete with physicians in terms of patient care or show competence in other areas, as we still need others to show us how.
5. To establish support systems for nursing, but do not organize effectively for work tasks. Do what's best for everyone, don't say what you mean, don't let people know what you want, and mostly be silent and noncommittal.[4]

Nurses are taught to "suggest" rather than "tell" and to chart "seems to be" as opposed to "is." Nurse educators who do practice and teach their students creativity, accountability, and assertiveness unfortunately send them to practice in institutions that continue to encourage and reward passivity and blind obedience.

Student nurses have been taught that as nurses, they have a designated role as professionals with professional rights and responsibilities. However, upon graduation they face reality shock in a profession full of inconsistencies where they are forbidden to function as professionals. What professional role is learned and what practicing role is expected rests with the clinical faculty and the hospital inservice educator. The nurse educator has a great responsibility to the student and to the nursing profession to help new nurses bridge the gap between education and service. One of the most effective ways is to learn to be assertive as a student.

It cannot be assumed that all nursing educators are assertive or understand the principles of assertion. The nurse educator may be assertive with students in the classroom but may not demonstrate assertion in the clinical area or in nursing practice. Appendix 9–A presents a test for evaluating assertiveness.

Of course, the assertiveness self-test, because of its lack of risk, allows for more assertive behavior than would the same situations in a clinical setting. Assertiveness training courses and readings such as those suggested at the end of this chapter can help in developing and sharpening assertive techniques.

For the remainder of this chapter, it will be assumed that the nurse educator can function assertively and is aware of the underlying principles of assertive behavior. The assertive educator has developed these skills through practice and by growth with a positive self-concept. The nurse who has self-respect as a person and as a professional can expect respect from others and receive it.

Certainly, students cannot all be expected or required to be assertive as an entry requirement. However, just as progression in nursing competence is required of students perhaps progressive competence in assertion and ultimately accountability should be expected. The nursing curriculum should include content whereby the student can learn about self and values. If it does not include assertiveness training, then the students should be encouraged to pursue it independently. Bibliographies and lists of courses should be provided for students. Chenevert's book, *STAT—Special Techniques in Assertiveness Training,* is an enjoyable, readable guideline that is especially designed for nurses.[5]

The educator who wishes to discuss assertiveness and risk taking with students can use supplemental handouts with definitions and examples and can assign required readings. Students should begin to explore their own feelings and behaviors outside the clinical area, categorizing their self-observations and feelings in a weekly log like the one shown in Exhibit 9–4. The objective of the weekly log is self-understanding. Students will begin to recognize their own attributes and gain self-respect. They can share their respective logs privately with the instructor, either verbally or in writing. Through dialogue the instructor can help the student identify nonassertive behavior. Destructive effects of this behavior should be discussed as well as areas where it might have been risky to use assertive behavior.

Gradually, students should be encouraged to assert themselves in low-risk situations (as when shopping in department stores). One-time encounters are

Exhibit 9–4 Student's Weekly Log

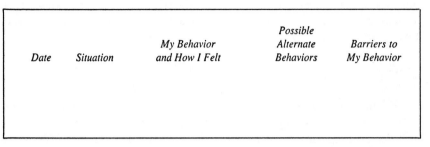

Date	Situation	My Behavior and How I Felt	Possible Alternate Behaviors	Barriers to My Behavior

usually safer for initial assertion than encounters with friends or relatives. Students' behavior should progress in assertiveness to high-risk situations. The readings required should give the student the information needed to observe the characteristic behavior of peers, instructors, staff members, physicians, and other health team members. Students should be able to identify the observed behavior as assertive, nonassertive, and aggressive, and to define the actions recorded in their own weekly journals, offering alternatives when appropriate.

A student activity for learning how to establish goals and take action assertively can be incorporated into the learning process. Students are asked to identify a problem area in their personal lives that requires resolution. By using the planning assertion form (Appendix 9–B) they can take the steps needed to find a solution using assertiveness techniques and skills. After completing the form, they can refer to the problem analysis guideline for problem situations encountered daily (Exhibit 9–5).

Most nursing programs have developed specific clinical objectives for each clinical experience; these focus on learning key principles in a variety of settings. The instructor can incorporate discussion of assertiveness in conjunction with clinical objectives. Pre- and post-conferences would include such discussion if objectives relating to student assertiveness were added to the curriculum's concep-

Exhibit 9–5 Guidelines for Problem Analysis

- What is the problem?
- Who/what is responsible for the problem?
- How have you contributed to the problem?
- What are the options to reduce or eliminate the problem?
- What are the advantages and risks of each option?

tual framework. If conference time is too limited for students to discuss their clients as they relate to the weekly focuses as well as to assess their own behavior with regard to assertiveness, they can have this dialogue with the instructor privately via the weekly journal.

ROLE PLAYING

Role playing is an excellent teaching and learning strategy in assertiveness training. It provides an opportunity for students to utilize assertiveness skills in a low-risk environment. It also allows students an avenue to vent their fantasies, frustrations, and fears concerning assertion. For example, "If I say that to her, she will say _____ and then I will _____." Role playing is especially good for venting the frustration or anger caused by stressful daily encounters. A group of students can review a stressful happening, examining what was said and what was not said. Feelings concerning the situation can be explored.

The role playing should take the following structure: the involved student explains the situation to the group, then plays himself or herself while another student assumes the role of the other involved party. After role playing the encounter, the students reverse roles and replay the encounter. The reversal allows the involved student to act out in a safe and risk-free environment any fears and fantasies about what could happen. It is by verbalizing the fears and acknowledging the fantasies that the student can logically deal with each irrational belief. Reversing roles a second time, the involved student resumes the original role but, having acted out hidden fears, can now deal more effectively with the situation should it occur. In most situations, students find their fears and projections to be completely irrational and totally unrealistic. Resuming the original role after role reversal usually produces more realistic actions and assertiveness skills.

Time should be provided for at least one role-playing session for each group while groups are learning assertion. Role playing can be engaged in on a one-to-one basis by instructor and student in a private conference, if necessary. Private sessions would allow students a more personal experience in an even less-threatening atmosphere than the group. By providing time for private role-playing sessions, the instructor conserves post-conference time for fulfilling clinical objectives. Exhibit 9–6 is an example of a role-playing situation.

Time should be allotted for the participants or other students to continue the dialogue if they wish. Not only will assertive behavior be reinforced in the involved students, but positive interaction among all participants will occur. Students should also be encouraged to express their concerns and strongest fears in these sessions. Irrational and fearful beliefs can be dispelled by mutual sharing among participants. Throughout the course the instructor must help each student determine which feelings and behaviors are assertive, which nonassertive, and which aggressive.

Exhibit 9–6 Role-Playing Exercise

In post-conference a student (A) tells the group about a client's pain and lack of relief from prescribed pain medication. The student has not asked the doctor to change the medication because of fear of how the doctor might respond to the questioning of orders.

Role-Playing Instructions: Approach the physician and make your request.

Student A: "Doctor, I am caring for Ms. J. and she is receiving Demerol 50 mg. q3h. for pain. After two hours, she is complaining of pain again. I would like you to consider changing the dosage or shortening the interval of the medication."

Student B: "Well, I really think she is getting enough, but we'll try 75 mg. q3h." (As the doctor, Student B may say anything.)

Role-Playing Instructions: Reverse roles.

Student B: (Repeat same request just made by Student A.)

Student A: "Who do you think you are prescribing medication? (Raising voice) I am the doctor and you are only a student nurse. Do you want to make the client an addict?"

Student B: (The student is given an opportunity to respond. Often in the initial role-playing experience, the student has no response or cannot respond to such an attack. In that case the instructor assumes the role.)

Instructor: (Assuming the role of the student nurse) "I understand that you are the doctor, but my responsibility is to report the client's response to your prescribed treatment. The client has been in pain for three days now and may have developed a drug tolerance, making the prescribed dose less effective."

THE ASSERTIVE ROLE MODEL

Educators must demonstrate assertive skills regularly in all areas of their personal and professional life. The risks involved are as high as the individual perceives them to be. A great deal of risk taking may be involved in communication with members of the health team from cooperating agencies. The relationship of the clinical instructor and the cooperating agency should be one of mutual respect. When disagreement occurs, it should be dealt with openly and honestly. When the instructor and a representative of the agency meet to discuss priorities prior to the arrival of the students for clinical practice, the educator should make clear that a major objective of the students' experience will be the development of personal and professional accountability through assertiveness. It is vital that the nurse educator establish a very positive dialogue with the health agency from the very beginning. If the situation is less than ideal the instructor must deal honestly and assertively with every issue. It may be prudent to intervene for the students at first and then help them progress gradually to active assertiveness as the clinical experience continues.

Some situations exist where the risk is too high to warrant assertiveness. These situations vary according to the educator's relationship with the staff and doctors. An instructor assigned to a new clinical area must enter each situation carefully, evaluating the positive and negative sides of the learning experiences available before deciding whether assertiveness would be productive.

When the educator chooses not to be assertive the reason should be shared with all the involved parties. Consider a situation like this:

> As a newly hired instructor assigned to a pediatric floor you are told that the head nurse has refused for years to allow student nurses to give medications to the children. As instructor you can choose one of the following courses of action:
>
> 1. Accept and continue the no-medication policy.
> 2. Continue the no-medication policy for the semester. Inform the head nurse that you will meet to discuss the situation and a resolution for the next semester.
> 3. Meet with the head nurse to discuss why this decision was made. Utilizing this information, try to work out with the head nurse an alternative course of action. Honestly share with the head nurse the impact of the no-medication policy on the learning of students.

The instructor must evaluate the "go along with" situations morally, ethically, and legally. He or she must consider the risks involved. In the preceding situation, the third alternative would be the most productive and allow for open and honest communications among the parties involved. Consider the next situation:

> Mr. S. is a 62-year-old male admitted for a cholecystectomy. During surgery metastatic cancer was found. Because of the extent, no surgical intervention was done. Post-operatively Mr. S. is undergoing an array of diagnostic studies to locate the primary site of the cancer. He is also receiving chemotherapy at the same time. The student tells you that Mr. S. does not know his diagnosis or why he is having all these tests. He could not tell the student what drugs he was receiving and why. The staff on the floor assure you that he has been told and that he is in "denial." The student continues to believe that the client does not understand and plans nursing care of the client with this in mind.

What are the risks in this situation if the student encourages the client to ask questions? What are the risks if the student does not? It seems that if nurses are professionally accountable, then they must accept the risks of professional confrontation for their clients' welfare. Can nurses continue to hide behind the claim "It's not my responsibility"?

Risk taking is an important component of assertiveness. Each risk situation must be evaluated on the basis of its relationship to quality nursing care and effective clinical instruction. Nurse educators are confronted with risk situations very frequently during the process of clinically instructing students. How they handle such situations may influence the risk-taking ability of their students in future interactions.

Effective assertive behavior is built on the key concept of personal power. Personal power, in this context, is defined as an internal strength that can influence the thoughts and/or actions of another. Coupled with this inner strength is the willingness and ability to interact with others to promote change. Nurse educators must fully develop their personal powers in order to interact assertively with others. It is only after nurse educators have refined their own personal powers that they can begin to cultivate personal power in nursing students. The following are some guidelines for personal power:

- Expect respect.
- Do not invite victimization.
- Cultivate your worth in your own eyes.
- Dress for success.
- Take the initiative to make relationships better.
- Practice honesty; avoid lies.
- Avoid waiting for things to get better.
- Give and accept criticism in a clear, straightforward manner.
- Build your own support systems.
- Maintain your control.
- Expect and give rewards for efforts.
- Accept mistakes in yourself and others.
- Eliminate unproductive complaining; act on your complaints.
- Evaluate your right to refuse in light of your responsibilities.
- Understand that assertive requesting will guarantee consideration (not always the results you want).
- Delight in your own humanness.
- Be your own best friend!

Nurse educators should demonstrate assertiveness and personal power in their nursing and educational practices. If this is accomplished, they can be an effective role model for nursing students and professional nurses.

SUMMARY

The importance of incorporating assertiveness training as part of clinical instruction can be measured only by the resulting behavior of involved students. The nurse educator should recognize the value of assertion in the curriculum and proceed in the manner suggested in this chapter. What must be remembered is that assertiveness can be taught only by someone who can demonstrate it personally and professionally. Thus, it is imperative that the nurse educator wishing to integrate assertiveness into clinical instruction has mastered the necessary skills prior to teaching them.

NOTES

1. Marlene Grissum and R. Spengler, *Womanpower and Health Care* (Boston: Little, Brown, 1976), 7.

2. Lynn Z. Bloom, Karen Coburn, and Joan Pearlman, *The New Assertive Woman* (New York: Dell, 1975).

3. Diane K. Jervik and Ida M. Martinson, *Women in Stress: A Nursing Perspective* (New York: Appleton-Century-Crofts, 1979), 31–32.

4. Sonya J. Herman, *Becoming Assertive: A Guide for Nurses* (New York: D. Van Nostrand, 1978), 125–126.

5. Melodie Chenevert, *STAT—Special Techniques in Assertiveness Training* (St. Louis: C.V. Mosby, 1983).

SUGGESTED READINGS

Alberti, R.E., and M.L. Emmons. *Your Perfect Right: A Guide to Assertive Behavior*, 2nd ed. San Luis Obispo, Calif.: Impact, 1974.

Ashley, J. *Hospitals, Paternalism and the Role of the Nurse*. New York: Teachers College Press, 1977.

Baer, Jean. *How To Be an Assertive (not Aggressive) Woman in Life, in Love, and on the Job*. New York: New American Library, 1976.

Bakdash, D. "Becoming an Assertive Nurse." *American Journal of Nursing* (October 1978): 1710–1712.

Bloom, L., K. Coburn, and J. Pearlman. *The New Assertive Woman*. New York: Dell, 1976.

Clark, Carolyn Chambers. *Assertive Skills for Nurses*. Wakefield, Mass.: Contemporary, 1978.

Donnelly, G. "The Assertive Nurse." *Nursing '78* (January 1978): 65–69.

Herman, S. *Becoming Assertive/A Guide for Nurses*. New York: D. Van Nostrand, 1978.

Newman, Mildred, and Bernard Berkowitz. *How To Be Your Own Best Friend*. New York: Ballantine, 1971.

Appendix 9–A

Assertiveness Test

SECTION A

Directions: Choose the answer that would best describe your behavior. Write the appropriate number on a separate sheet. Be sure to answer every question. The scoring directions at the end of the test show you how to evaluate your own responses.

1. A client is receiving Demerol 50 mg q3h for incisional pain. It is the evening of his surgery. After 2 hours, the client is c/o again. You tell the head nurse that he probably needs a larger dose. The head nurse, whom you respect, tells you that the particular doctor will not change the order. What do you do?

   a. Tell the student that if you were head nurse, you would call the doctor.
   b. Tell the student that you will call the doctor.
   c. Instruct the student to approach the physician when he arrives.
   d. Instruct the student to leave the matter to the head nurse.

2. The physician has written an order "Do not allow client to smoke because of cardiac condition." The client, well informed of the implications, asks your student for a match. What do you do?

   a. Give the client a match.
   b. Tell the client to get a match from someone else.
   c. Don't give the client the match, but tell the doctor that the client has the right to make a decision.
   d. Tell your student to inform the client why the student cannot provide the match.

201

3. A doctor writes on the order sheet: "Client is not to know diagnosis." Your student is assigned to this client. The client asks the student about the diagnosis. The student approaches you and you say

   a. Inform the doctor of the client's desire to know.
   b. Tell the client you really do not know.
   c. You will discuss the issue with the physician before informing the client.
   d. You tell the client what is wrong.
   e. Inform the head nurse and have the head nurse talk to the doctor.

4. You recommend an intervention for a family in crisis in a clinical pre-conference. All the students except one agree with you. The one student is adamant and disagrees openly and offers an alternative. You

   a. Indicate that you respect the student's opinion, but that your intervention is more appropriate.
   b. Ask why the student feels more qualified to recommend an intervention.
   c. Listen to the student and ask others to comment on both recommendations.
   d. Listen to the student, then direct the conference to another topic.

5. Your student has not ambulated the client as ordered. The physician, upon discovering this, proceeds to scream at the student in the hall. You

   a. Role play with the student in post-conference how to handle such encounters in the future.
   b. Remind the student about the hazards of immobility.
   c. Have the student accompany you to inform the physician that the emotional display was unacceptable.
   d. Discuss this in post-conference.
   e. Report the doctor's unacceptable behavior to the head nurse.

SECTION B

Directions: On a scale of 1 to 6, 1 representing *Always* and 6 representing *Never*, circle the appropriate number.

1. When in a conflict situation, I tell students that "If I was
   charge nurse, I would . . ."   6 5 4 3 2 1
2. I am a passive person.   6 5 4 3 2 1
3. I am a passive nurse.   6 5 4 3 2 1
4. I am an aggressive person.   6 5 4 3 2 1

5. I am an aggressive nurse.   6 5 4 3 2 1
6. When a student openly challenges me, I am openly upset.   6 5 4 3 2 1

Total points   _____

SCORING

Directions: Total the point values of each of the responses you chose that best describes your behavior in each situation:

Situation 1: a = 2, b = 3, c = 4, d = 1.
Situation 2: a = 4, b = 1, c = 3, d = 2.
Situation 3: a = 4, b = 2, c = 5, d = 1, e = 3.
Situation 4: a = 3, b = 2, c = 4, d = 1.
Situation 5: a = 4, b = 2, c = 5, d = 1, e = 3.

Add the total points: Section A _____ + Section B _____ = TOTAL TEST POINTS _____

If your total points range from

56 to 40 you have demonstrated a pattern of assertive behavior.

39 to 18 you have demonstrated a tendency to fluctuate between assertive and nonassertive behavior. In actual situations you probably would demonstrate a nonassertive pattern.

17 to 6 you have demonstrated a pattern of nonassertive behavior.

Appendix 9–B

Assertiveness Planning

Assertiveness is a learned behavior that involves step-by-step change in behavior patterns. The following exercise will help you establish goals and explore possible outcomes

A. List the changes you would like to make in your private life.
B. List the changes you would like to make in your professional life.
C. Review the changes you have listed and select the two most important to you. Rewrite them as goals.
1. Personal goals
   a.
   b.
2. Professional goals
   a.
   b.
D. Complete this chart

Goals	What is blocking you from pursuing each goal?	What behavior changes are needed by you to achieve your goals?	What resources (person, agencies) can assist you to attain your goals?
Personal			
1.			
2.			
Professional			
1.			
2.			

E. List the specific actions needed to achieve each of your personal and professional goals. Set a timetable for each action.

Goals	Specific actions	Timetable Onset of actions	Achievement of goals
Personal			
1.			
2.			
Professional			
1.			
2.			

Chapter 10

Leadership and Clinical Instruction

Many important issues have come and gone in nursing in recent times, but one that continues to be addressed is whether nursing is a profession. The question of whether nursing encompasses the attributes of a profession becomes relevant when one analyzes the role of the professional nurse. The characteristics that are demonstrated by the group members are usually the basis for determining professionalism. In discussing this concept, Styles introduces a new term called *professionhood*, which "focuses on the characteristics of the individual as a member of a profession," as opposed to *professionalism*, which "emphasizes the composite character of the profession."[1] Professionhood emphasizes individual responsibility as opposed to passivism or blamism.

Certain themes seem to surface as one examines the list of criteria used to denote a professional person. According to Styles these include:

- service commitment
- ethical behavior
- a particular expertise
- a particular body of scientific knowledge
- extensive university education
- collegiality of members
- autonomy in setting standards of education and practice[2]

Of these characteristics, personal and professional autonomy is the most applicable to leadership in nursing. "Autonomy" is defined by Webster's unabridged dictionary as "self-governing, without outside control."[3] Autonomy in nursing practice and education is vital to the survival of nursing and its quest for professionalism.

Autonomy and power in nursing can be cultivated by individual professional nurses in service and education. By practicing nursing excellence, nurses can demonstrate to society that professional nursing is essential for high-quality health care. The difference that professional nursing can make in the quality of health care received by the consumer could do more to foster autonomy in the nursing profession than all other possible strategies for change.

Autonomy and leadership in nursing cannot be separated. It is through the development of personal autonomy of the individual nurse that nursing can become autonomous. The profession's autonomy would be reflected in its leadership in the health care delivery system.

Leadership and management skills are a group of behaviors that influence individuals and groups of individuals (see Figure 10–1). This behavior encourages others toward specific outcomes determined desirable by the leader.

A leader is instrumental in assisting peers, superiors, and subordinates to attain agency, professional, and personal goals. Achievement of effective leadership and management skills is as important for the staff nurse as for the head nurse or supervisor. All nurses are leaders and managers whether they are in nursing service or education. Students of professional nursing should be given the opportunity to discover the principles of management and leadership.

Most nursing programs offer some type of leadership or management courses for professional nurses. Such courses usually cover the theory of management, yet most lack practical experience—concurrent clinical experience in which to practice leadership skills. Case studies and role playing in clinical leadership may be effective teaching strategies, but they should not be used exclusively. Interactions must be provided also to give students the opportunity to apply classroom principles to clinical practice.

In nursing programs where the leadership course is an elective or not required at all, the nurse educator will have to incorporate the theory and practice into the clinical courses. If no classroom time is allotted for leadership theory, then a creative educator can devote some conference time to it. Focus sheets are effective for learning these skills (see Exhibit 10–1). Since all the students cannot be the leader at the same time, they can alternate the experience.

Figure 10–1 Components of Leadership

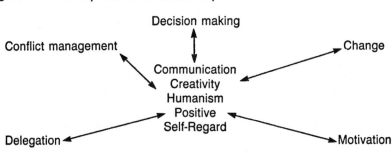

Exhibit 10–1 Clinical Focus Sheet for Leadership

FOCUS: Management experience

OBJECTIVES: The learner is expected to do the following:

A. Read assigned articles on leadership and management skills prior to experience.

B. Prepare assignments
  1. Review the charts of the assigned client population.
  2. Rank important data according to priority for use in providing client care.
  3. Identify members of the nursing team and read their job descriptions if needed. The educational preparation of each staff member should be considered.
  4. Clients are assigned according to their needs (physical, psychosocial, treatments, and learning) to the personnel best prepared to care for them.
  5. Other criteria can also be considered if pertinent and known (preferences of staff and clients, age, maturity, experience, etc.).
  6. Information needed on the assigned sheet
    a. Client names and room numbers
    b. Specific duties (such as assisting another staff member)
    c. Lunch and break times with name of relief person
  7. Miscellaneous
    a. Assign empty beds in case of new admissions
    b. Assign clients close together if possible
    c. Consider the amount of time each client requires instead of just the total number of assigned clients

C. Give personnel assignments individually. The amount of detail will be dependent on the level of experience of the personnel. Post assignment in a central location.

D. Acquire data for shift report (see Exhibit 10–2).

E. Evaluate your management experience during your weekly student self-evaluation.

MANAGEMENT AND LEADERSHIP

During the clinical experience focused on leadership, the learner should function as nursing manager. He or she must be held accountable for the clinical learning objectives and for the functions of the manager's position. The educator must share the objectives with the head nurse. Open dialogue is vital to the success of this learning experience. The learner's assignment should consist of approximately one-third to one-half the floor population, 10 to 12 clients being the ideal number. If too large a group of clients is assigned, the situation may end in chaos, with the student or new graduate feeling frustrated over an unsuccessful try at leadership.

If at all possible the learner should be required to participate in preclinical planning sessions the day before the assigned clinical experience. While other students are assessing the needs of their clients according to the nursing process, the student manager should become informed about clients and staff. A joint planning session should be arranged with the head nurse in order to coordinate the learning experiences of the student leader and the management operations of the clinical unit. Input from the head nurse would assist the student to establish criteria for making assignments for the following day.

If a preclinical planning session cannot be held beforehand, the student will have to gather the information, establish priorities of care, and make assignments the same day as the clinical experience. Usually one-half to one hour of time is needed to complete this important task of client need assessment and assignment making. Interaction between head nurse and the student manager must be encouraged for this experience to be an effective learning experience. After discussing ideas with the head nurse and obtaining information, the student should attend shift report and then readjust his or her priorities and assignments accordingly. After report the student manager must meet with each staff member individually to discuss the assignment for the day and to assist in planning care for the assigned clients.

The student already has a theoretical base for these activities and so can proceed to complete this portion of the leadership task with minimal assistance from the nurse educator. After completing the assigned readings on the subject, the student should demonstrate knowledge about the criteria for making assignments and need guidance only occasionally. This would not prevent the educator from being utilized as a resource person, however; nor would it prohibit periodic critiques of the student's performance.

The educator should encourage the student manager to utilize walking rounds in assigning clients to the staff personnel. *Walking rounds* is an information-gathering strategy wherein the charge nurse and the staff member visit the clients at bedside. This accomplishes two purposes in the leadership experience for the learner: the student manager can (1) assess the client's condition on the spot and explain client care and any changes with the assigned staff member and (2) identify pertinent information necessary to establish priorities of the shift.

DECISION MAKING

An effective leader or professional is one who can arrive at accurate decisions. The accuracy of the decision is influenced by the ability of the nurse to:

- recognize cues
- validate inferences

- generate options
- select appropriate or effective options

The recognition of cues and the interpretation of the cues leads to validated inferences. This is a complex cognitive process that is strongly influenced by the quality and quantity of stored patterns of knowledge. In other words, one cannot notice or attach meaning to a cue that one doesn't know. Thus, if the nurse does not know the signs and symptoms of increased intracranial pressure, he or she will not notice early cues.

After the cues have been interpreted or meaning attached to them, the nurse has several options to choose from:

- do nothing
- monitor
- collect more data
- consult or collaborate
- delegate
- refer to another
- intervene directly

Decision making in the leadership experience occurs throughout the clinical practice session. Gathering client information, establishing priorities of care, and making assignments all involve important decisions by the student manager.

Although the student manager should have a chance to make most decisions, because of the variety of problems that could arise, the following options should be available:

- Make the decision, but discuss it with the nurse educator prior to acting.
- Offer two or three alternatives for discussion with the nurse educator.
- If a decision is needed quickly, experienced personnel will proceed, but the student should make a decision and share it retrospectively.

The nurse educator can explore with the student each decision and the options available. A prudent educator should caution the student manager against any particular choice where failure can be predicted. However, to encourage creativity students should be permitted to follow through with their decisions whenever possible.

The student manager's experience should culminate with an in-depth report on the client population at the end of the shift. This would involve evaluating data collected by the assigned unit personnel for relevancy (see Exhibit 10–2 for guidelines). The report for the next shift should omit unimportant and irrelevant

Exhibit 10–2 Guidelines for Shift Report

A brief and concise report is to be given. For each client this report should include:

1. Client's name, diagnosis, age, and physician.
2. General condition and special needs. Allergies, previous history, if pertinent.
3. Special changes over last 16 hours.
4. Problems or potential difficulties.
5. Significant medication or treatment information, i.e., reactions, blood administration, anticoagulant therapy.
6. Pending discharges and/or transfers.
7. Schedules for today. For example, OR, tests, diagnostic procedures, consultations, physical therapy, dialysis (including time if known).
8. Information essential to proper care and coordination of service and operation of unit.
9. Intravenous therapy, drainages. Total intake and output on critical patients.

information in order to provide a clear and concise description of the client population and care. After the experience, the student should evaluate the learning experience and decisions as directed in the leadership focus sheet (Exhibit 10–1).

The inservice educator can utilize the same teaching strategies to assist new graduates to develop leadership skills. Offering the new nurses information about delegation, decision making, and assignment making through lecture, audiovisual aids, or assigned readings will provide them with the theoretical basis for attaining leadership skills. The new graduate's experience related to assignment and decision making can proceed in the same order and by the same method as that of the student learner. The inservice educator can function in the same roles as the nurse educator who works with the student manager.

The inservice educator must also lay the groundwork for this leadership experience by sharing the objectives and content of the experience with the head nurse. Meetings between the inservice educator, the graduate, and the head nurse would establish a basis for the learner's performance and identify the framework within which the graduate should function. Close supervision and guidance by the inservice educator will provide support and direction during the process of developing and applying leadership and management skills.

CONFLICT MANAGEMENT

Conflict management is a technique of leadership that enables the professional nurse to intervene constructively with superior, peers, subordinates, and clients and their families. Conflict can be described as the tension produced whenever interdependent individuals disagree about important issues.[4] Thus, conflict management is the act of assertively dealing with the tensions that have accumulated as the result of strong disagreements. How a nurse leader handles conflict can determine the effectiveness of his or her leadership and management.

Conflict is inherent in all interaction when there is more than one opinion expressed about a topic. But whether the resolution is constructive or destructive depends on the individual actions of the persons involved. Exhibit 10–3 shows that conflict is neutral and natural but can become either destructive or constructive according to the strategies selected by the involved persons to deal with the conflict.

Certain conflicts are unique to the nursing profession. Kramer and Schmalenberg identified them as

- Goals vs. means conflict
- Competency gap conflict
- Professional vs. bureaucratic conflict
- Expressive vs. instrumental
- Differential role expectation conflicts
  - Nurse vs. nurse
  - Nurse vs. client
  - Nurse vs. physician
- Competing roles[5]

These researchers subscribe to the belief that constructive resolution of conflict can be achieved by identifying the sources of conflict.

Exhibit 10–3 Characteristics of Conflict

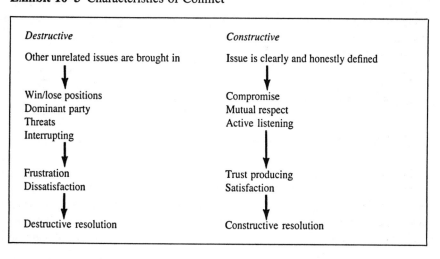

The goals versus means conflict arises out of the belief that a nurse's primary function is to assist the client in getting well. This is true; nonetheless in certain clinical situations the client will not get well. So the nurse has a conflict between the projected goal and the reality of the situation.

The professional versus bureaucratic conflict results from the nurses' realization that tne system that employs them often has different goals than theirs. School has .aught nurses to expect certain situations, yet now they are faced with very different ones.

New graduates experience competency gap conflicts when they find their own performance does not meet their perceived standards of nursing. The inexperienced nurse who is assigned clients who require extensive physical care will need more time than experienced nurses. However, a conflict may arise because of the additional time needed or because of care that may have to be omitted due to lack of time.

Differential role expectation conflicts occur when a nurse's expectations for a situation differ from another nurse's, a physician's, or the client's. Examples of this conflict are a physician's refusal to tell a client a diagnosis or a client's demands for attention that are unrealistic for a nurse's workload.

Expressive function versus instrumental conflicts are created when the nurse is caught between meeting the unique human needs of the clients and getting tasks done. More conflict often arises when the nurse chooses one over the other.

The competing roles conflict is characteristic of nurses who also have responsibilities as spouses or parents. Too often the responsibilities of nursing deplete one physically and mentally, leaving little energy for personal life.

To help learners with nursing conflicts, the assignment presented in Exhibit 10–4 can be utilized.

Recognizing the sources of conflict will not resolve them, but it helps to know that certain conflicts are inherent to nursing. Besides knowing in what areas to

---

Exhibit 10–4 Assignment: Managing Conflict

Read "Conflict: The Cutting Edge of Growth," by M. Kramer and C. Schmalenberg, *The Journal of Nursing Administration* (October 1976): 19–25.

Give an example of a conflict *that you have experienced* as a nurse and place it in the appropriate category. Find at least one example for each category.

1. Professional/bureaucratic
2. Personal competency gap
3. Differential self/other role expectations
4. Means/goal
5. Expressive/instrumental
6. Competing roles

anticipate problems, one should be aware which conflicts can be resolved, which reduced, and most important, which *cannot* be resolved. Conflicts can often be reduced to a manageable size if the type can be identified.

Conflicts of an interpersonal nature can be dealt with successfully by means of the assertiveness techniques discussed in Chapter 9. Conflict need not have a negative outcome; with effort a constructive resolution can be achieved.

CHANGE THEORY

To *change* means, according to Webster, "to alter by substituting something else for or by giving up for something else."[6] Nurses and nursing have been and always will be continuously facing change. Most nurses would agree that change is necessary to meet the demands of technology, society, and the profession for the improvement of the health care delivery system. How changes are perceived and implemented depends on the process, the rate, and the agent of change. Resistance to change is expected but can be minimized when change is planned.

Change theory can be integrated into a traditional clinical course, as are other nontraditional topics, like assertiveness. The instructor can devise a focus sheet with assigned readings and case study analysis. A written assignment like that in Exhibit 10–5 might be useful as well.

Students discussing change often fail to recognize how they can be agents of change. Nursing education teaches students idealism about client care, and nursing service teaches them realism—about the realities of nursing they will encounter after graduation. Students are dismayed by the vast differences between theory and practice. They complain about the quality of care administered to the client and about the nonnursing tasks delegated to nurses.

The nurse educator should acknowledge the differences but should not encourage purposeless complaining and grumbling. Instead, the clinical instructor should help students apply creative problem solving to specific concerns and incorporate appropriate strategies for change into the clinical experience. Students as well as educators must realize that most change comes about very slowly. Students who can witness productive change within a health care system will be better equipped to function as change agents after graduation.

Exhibit 10–5 Assignment: Managing Change

1. Identify a change that you believe is needed on the unit or in the agency where you work.
2. Identify the factors that may cause resistance to your proposed change.
3. What could be done to reduce these factors?

In the following example creative problem solving is applied in change intervention:

> Some students complained that clients on a skilled care facility were bored and spent most of their day sleeping. Together they brainstormed a variety of nursing interventions. After considering the advantages and disadvantages of each alternative, they chose one.
>
> The students chose to provide the clients with a place for community dining. Since the facility had such a room, the only barrier to this proposal was convincing the staff that the difficulty of having to help immobile clients to the dining room was outweighed by the outcome.
>
> The students proposed that on the two days each week when they were there the client could choose to eat in the dining room. On those days the students kept a record of the amount of food consumed and daytime sleeping. Clients were also observed for other changes. The staff were persuaded to keep a similar record on the other days, when the clients ate in their rooms.
>
> After two weeks the staff reported that clients looked forward to the days that they ate in the dining room. Food consumption greatly increased (it almost doubled), and the amount of daytime sleeping decreased. Other changes observed on days the dining room was used were that clients remained in the dining room talking after meals, clients slept better at night without sedation, and clients took interest in their dress and grooming.
>
> As a consequence, the staff not only began providing regular dining room service for all meals, but also planned a recreational activity followed by a snack three times a week.

The inservice educator too must guide new leaders. The shock of entering the real world of health care can discourage and overwhelm the new graduate who does not receive support and encouragement. The ideals the new nurse has incorporated into professional life patterns must be encouraged by the educator, who should also demonstrate how to function effectively in the real nursing world. Without this support the new graduate may become disheartened and dissatisfied and choose to leave the profession; new graduates who stay often discard idealistic values and fall into routine nursing that incorporates qualities previously despised. Educators should be cautious, however, not to imply to students or new graduates that they will be able to make major changes in any system. Newcomers to any system must first be accepted as members before changes they propose are considered. The empathetic inservice educator can assist the graduate to make the necessary adjustments while still maintaining the high standards learned in nursing school. Once established and adjusted, the nurse can proceed to act as a change agent in the health care system, demonstrating the leadership and management skills needed to reinforce the autonomy of the nursing profession.

DELEGATION

Delegation of responsibility means directing a subordinate or peer to perform a task for which one is responsible. Most nurses have difficulty delegating responsibility because they view it as telling others to do something that they could do themselves. The failure of the nurse leader to delegate wastes money for the institution and time and effort for the professional nurse.

A head nurse who carries out a task that should be delegated to another nurse is wasting agency money (the difference between the head nurse's salary and that of the person who should be carrying out the function) and wasting valuable time that should be devoted to supervisory activities. Every time an action is not delegated properly, time is spent needlessly, and areas where the head nurse's expertise is needed are left unattended.

The educator must instruct students in delegation of appropriate tasks to appropriate persons very early in the nursing program. Students should be encouraged to have ward secretaries make phone calls to various departments and have nonprofessionals provide transport and errand services. The educator must explain to the nurse leader on the unit the principles behind these actions at the joint conference held prior to the students' entrance on the unit. This will encourage the staff to evaluate their own actions related to delegation of professional and nonprofessional activities, as well as provide them with an explanation of why students "will not" make their own phone calls and "will not" take lab slips to hematology.

Establishing the groundwork prior to the students' experience on the unit will encourage open dialogue between nursing service and nursing education. It may also be a first step toward change on a unit where delegation is virtually nonexistent. The inservice educator should encourage both experienced staff and new graduates to delegate responsibility appropriately.

Often nurses believe that it is easier to complete tasks themselves than to explain them in detail to others. However, if delegation is not effectively carried out on a unit, the staff will fail to grow in experience and knowledge. The entire staff should be provided with new and different opportunities for learning. If the nurse leader fails to delegate, the staff's educational process will be stifled and the quality of the care provided to the client will suffer.

Delegation requires planning, teaching, and evaluating. Students who are learning leadership and management skills must also learn how to delegate responsibility to others; Volante lists three steps:

1. Define the tasks you want done.
2. Relay the task, time limit, and expected results.
3. Establish controls and checkpoints.[7]

The educator should help the student determine how much information needs to be passed along to the persons to whom responsibility is to be delegated. Some people need only a verbal definition of a task, whereas others would need explicit written directions for the same task. An example of delegation to different levels of staff follows:

> *To a professional nurse:* Please get Ms. Black out of bed for the first time this morning.
>
> *To a nursing assistant:* Ms. Black needs to be dangled. Evaluate her color and comfort before getting her up. If these are acceptable, help her to a chair three feet from the bed. Please ask for assistance if you are unsure of her condition.

The inservice educator can teach the same principles of delegation to staff and new graduates. Readings and other information can be provided prior to their attempts at delegation and, again, support and supervision will be required.

SUMMARY

Professional nurses and nursing students must believe that they have special skills and knowledge to function as leaders in nursing. They must free themselves from traditions that have historically prevented nurses from advancing their profession.

Clinical instructors should not only teach all aspects of leadership but also be leaders themselves. Serving as a role model is the best way to teach leadership. Moreover, professional nurse educators should use all management and leadership skills at their disposal to bring about the changes that are so badly needed if nursing is to grow as a vital health care profession. For, as Styles expressed it, ''the professionalism of nursing will be achieved only through the professionhood of its members.''[8]

NOTES

1. Margretta M. Styles, *On Nursing—Toward A New Endowment* (St. Louis: C.V. Mosby, 1982), 47.
2. Ibid., 8.
3. *Webster's Third New International Dictionary.*

4. Marlene Kramer and Claudia E. Schmalenberg, "Conflict: The Cutting Edge of Growth," *The Journal of Nursing Administration* (October 1976):19–25.

5. Ibid.

6. *Webster's Third New International Dictionary.*

7. Elena M. Volante, "Mastering the Managerial Skill of Delegation," *The Journal of Nursing Administration* (January–February 1974):25–27.

8. Styles, 47.

SUGGESTED READINGS

Cooper, J. "Conflict: How To Avoid It and What To Do When You Can't." *Nursing 79,* no. 9 (January 1979):89–91.

Diers, Donna. "Lessons on Leadership." *Image* 5 (October 1979):67–71.

Donnelly, G., A. Mengel, and D. Sutterly. *The Nursing System: Issues, Ethics, and Politics.* New York: John Wiley, 1980.

Douglass, Laura Mae. *The Effective Nurse—Leader and Manager.* St. Louis: C.V. Mosby, 1980.

Douglass, Laura Mae, and E.M. Olivia Bevis. *Nursing Management and Leadership in Action,* 3rd ed. St. Louis: C.V. Mosby, 1979.

Gale, Charlotte B. "Walking in the Aide's Shoes." *American Journal of Nursing* 73 (April 1973):612–613.

Kemp, V. "An Overview of Change and Leadership." *Topics in Clinical Nursing* 6 (April 1984):1–9.

Kramer, Marlene, and Claudia E. Schmalenberg. "Conflict: The Cutting Edge of Growth." *The Journal of Nursing Administration* 6 (October 1976):19–25.

Levi, Margaret. "Functional Redundancy and the Process of Professionalism: The Case of Registered Nurses in the United States." *Journal of Health Politics, Policy and Law* 3 (Summer 1980):333–348.

Marriner, A. "Conflict Theory." *Supervisor Nurse* 14 (October 1979):12–16.

———. "Conflict Resolution." *Supervisor Nurse* 14 (May 1979):46–56.

Mauksch, Ingeborg G., and Michael H. Miller. *Implementing Change in Nursing.* St. Louis: C.V. Mosby, 1981.

Myrtle, R., and E. Glogow. "How Nursing Administrators View Conflict." *Nursing Research* 27 (March–April 1978):103–106.

Nehls, D., et al. "Planned Change: A Quest for Nursing Autonomy." *The Journal of Nursing Administration* 4 (April 1974):23–27.

Partridge, K. "Nursing Values in a Changing Society." *Nursing Outlook* 26 (June 1978):356–360.

Plaszynski, L. "A Systematic Approach to Leadership Selection." *The Journal of Nursing Administration* 9 (March 1979):6–15.

Simeon, S.R. "Educators as Change Agents in the Institution of Nursing." *Journal of Continuing Education* 6 (June 1975):7–12.

Simms, L., and J. Lindberg. *The Nurse Person.* New York: Harper & Row, 1978.

Stevens, Barbara J. "Effecting Change." *The Journal of Nursing Administration* 5 (February 1975):23–26.

Sweeney, Mary Ann, et al. "Essential Skills for Baccalaureate Graduates: Perspectives of Education and Service." *The Journal of Nursing Administration* 8 (October 1980):37–44.

Volante, Elena M. "Mastering the Managerial Skill of Delegation." *The Journal of Nursing Administration* (January–February 1974):25–27.

Welch, L.B., ed. "The Nurse as a Change Agent." *Nursing Clinics in North America* 8 (1979):305–383.

Wiley, Loy. "Getting along Better with Those Aides." *Nursing 75*, no. 5 (1975):67–74.

———. "Shifting Smoothly." *Nursing 75*, no. 5 (1975):85–90.

Chapter 11

Evaluation and Clinical Instruction

Clinical evaluation has posed a challenge for nurse educators for many years. The term itself usually evokes an emotional response in both evaluators and learners. Students under evaluation dread the possible dredging up of every error made when they were novices functioning at their worst. Nurse educators, remembering their own experiences with student evaluations, often concentrate on being fair and just and giving the student the benefit of the doubt. But in the effort to make sure that each student is judged fairly, they may overlook potential and actual clinical incompetencies and nursing practices that are unsafe. To avoid this pitfall the nurse educator must base student evaluations upon objective competency-based criteria and not upon vague definitions of what makes a good or bad professional nurse.

Evaluation in the classroom is the process of determining a quantitative score based on predominately objective data. Evaluation in the clinical setting is the process of collecting data in order to make a judgment as applied to a standard or criteria. Clinical evaluation is a subjective conclusion made by an educator about objective performance or behavior. It cannot be a totally objective evaluation because the individual educator must render a judgment on such questions as:

- How many incidents warrant failure?
- What types of incidents warrant failure?
- How much improvement warrants passing?
- How much performance deficits can be permitted for anxiety?

GOALS OF EVALUATION

In nursing *evaluation* can be described as the process of gathering and analyzing data for the purpose of determining whether desired outcomes have been successfully achieved. For nursing educators it means determining whether students have met the objectives of the course, clinical experience, or the position.

The goals of clinical evaluation of the nursing student are

• To determine whether the student has sufficient knowledge for the established level of clinical practice.
• To provide feedback to discourage or encourage certain behavior.

A health agency must also utilize clinical evaluations to assess the performance of students and employees. In addition to the goals stated for students, two more must be included for clinical evaluation of nursing graduates:

• To determine the distribution of merit pay.
• To provide a record for the promotion, demotion, and dismissal of an employee.

CLINICAL TEACHING VERSUS EVALUATION

Because of the dilemmas that clinical evaluation represent to faculty and students, attempts have been made to separate evaluation time from teaching and practice time. An example of one such attempt is reserving two days at the end of a semester or period in which each student's performance is evaluated. This type of evaluation is often called summative by some educators. During the period prior to the two days, students are not evaluated. Unfortunately, this system has several drawbacks.

• It fundamentally depicts evaluation as a negative experience.
• It will probably not pass a student whose performance all period has been good but was unsatisfactory during the two-day period.
• It will probably pass a student whose performance all period was unsatisfactory but was satisfactory during the two-day period.

Perhaps the faculty need to closely examine why such a system is desired.

Clinical teaching and learning is a time for practice, for learning, and for evaluation. If evaluation is viewed as encouraging and discouraging certain behaviors, it is indeed an element in most faculty-student interactions. As students progress through the curriculum, they will be learning and practicing new knowledge and skills; however, they also will be evaluated on their past learning. For example, a student performing a urinary catheterization for the first time will not be evaluated on his or her ability to successfully catheterize or on his or her ability to remember the procedure since first-time experiences are very anxiety provoking. However, this student may be evaluated on past learning, e.g., knowledge of aseptic technique. Contaminating a catheter should not be evaluated as unsatisfactory unless the student fails to acknowledge the need to acquire a new catheter.

Prior to any supervised new experience, the student should be advised that he or she will not be evaluated on the unfamiliar skills and knowledge during this first encounter, only those of past learning experiences.

The conflict between the learner's needs and the need for evaluation is a major dilemma inherent in clinical instruction. The student must be provided with opportunities to practice and perfect skills but must function safely in the process. Educators often deliberately overlook unacceptable practices of a student who "has not had the time to practice the skill." It would be well for both student and educator to remember that evaluation is a fact of life. It will not disappear for the student upon graduation from the nursing program. It is a reality that in life one's professional performance is always evaluated by others. Students must realize that the quality of their performance in the clinical setting is important regardless of whether they are being directly evaluated or not. The educator has the responsibility to help the student learn from errors and not brush them off as irrelevant "because it is not evaluation time."

In an attempt to evolve the perfect evaluation tool that will stand the challenge of failing or unsatisfactory students faculty strive to design a *pure* objective evaluation system. The results are usually a lengthy detailed document. Despite the descriptive behavioral criteria, the individual faculty member still must render a subjective judgment on the ability or quality of the student's performance.

No evaluation tool can instill confidence and credibility for a faculty member, especially in situations with an unsatisfactory student. The confidence and credibility of an educator is fostered by the acquisition of:

- clinical expertise
- open, honest dialogue
- sound, caring counseling and coaching techniques
- sound documentation

The educational program, through the faculty, dean, or chairperson, can assist the educator in clinical evaluation by providing:

- academic policies that clearly indicate criteria for promotion and failure
- assistance for individual faculty members in the decision-making process, e.g., record keeping
- emotional support for individual faculty members during the process of a clinical failure

When one accepts a faculty position, one assumes that some students will not be able to meet the expected level of performance and that the responsibility to identify, coach, and sometimes fail a student is the faculty's. Sometimes faculty believe because their admission standards are high this will eliminate failing students. If one closely examines this belief, it proposes that an individual can be successful in nursing if he or she has an excellent academic record. However, nursing is a profession with both theoretical and practice components.

Benner describes expert clinical nurses as nurses who through repeated clinical encounters and theoretical understanding acquire skilled clinical knowledge. Skilled clinical knowledge is the learning that is acquired by applying theory to practice and by refining of preconceived theory.[1] Nurses who practice without a sound theoretical base are just as unskilled as nurses who practice without sound clinical skills. Benner concludes that one cannot be an expert nurse without clinical expertise, despite the number of letters after one's name.[2] Expertise comes only after repetitive clinical encounters where predictive clinical decision making is practiced. Thus educators should be able to predict that each student will be able to acquire clinical skills based on sound, refined theoretical knowledge.

Passing students knowing that they will fail as graduates either clinically or on state boards is a grave violation of one's professional standards. The professional obligation of "do no harm" is violated threefold, for those who will *suffer* will be the student, the clients, and ultimately the profession. Nursing is not a profession if it is not comprised of professionals. Specific strategies for the failing or unsatisfactory student are discussed at the end of this chapter.

PLANNING THE EVALUATION PROCESS

Prior to the evaluation of actual teaching-learning clinical experiences, the following should be considered in order to ensure effective, constructive clinical evaluations:

- Academic standards should be clearly documented, published, and revised periodically.
- The evaluation tool should be able to measure the learning of the content that has been identified as critical in the conceptual framework and course objectives.[3]
- The tool should progress with increasingly complex objectives culminating with the terminal objectives of the program.[4]
- The method of evaluation should be appropriate for the learning objectives being measured.
- The minimum standard of performance for the tool should be specified.

- The evaluation should be both formative and summative.
- The evaluation tool should be designed for multifaculty input when indicated.
- Designated periods for recording and sharing the evaluation process should be established.
- A detailed outline of the grievance procedure should be written and published in the student handbook.

Academic Standards

For too long nursing has been struggling to become recognized as a profession. This quest for professionalism has forced nursing to rise above those traits that identified it as an occupation and promote those attributes that will permit nursing to achieve professional status.

As high technology enters the health care system, nurses are expected to function at an extremely high level of proficiency. Their role has expanded to overlap that of the physician and to include knowledge that is quite sophisticated and complex. Nurses must be prepared to handle this change while assuming accountability for quality patient care. Nursing education is meeting the challenge by increasing the depth and breadth of knowledge presented in schools of nursing. Therefore, to be successful in nursing, individuals now entering nursing education must be of higher caliber than those previously admitted into nursing programs.

Another development affecting nursing is the depressed economic situation in the United States. As health care costs increase, fewer individuals are able to enter the health care delivery system for care. Hospital census have decreased dramatically which, in turn, have reduced the number of registered nurses needed by health care agencies. Thus, the nursing shortage that previously existed is now over. Within this context, it should be expected that only highly qualified registered nurses will find employment in the future.

The major responsibility of collegiate-based programs has been to prepare highly educated individuals who would demonstrate professional and technical competency in the practice of nursing. In order to clearly designate what constitutes professionally and technically competent practitioners of nursing, detailed policies should be developed that encompass the progression, retention, and graduation of nursing students. Such policies should include the following:

- course prerequisites
- incomplete grades
- grade point average requirement for nursing and non-nursing courses
- academic probation
- clinical probation
- academic dismissal

Measurement of Critical Learning

Faculty often develop lengthy evaluation tools in hope that the final judgment will require little subjectivity. Instead of creating a complex document to reflect a skill list, faculty should consider developing behavioral objectives that reflect critical concepts of the curriculum. A student must be successful in *every* objective since the objectives will represent only critical learning. Appendix 11–A presents a clinical evaluation based on critical elements.

Simple-to-Complex Learning Objectives

The tool that is used to evaluate clinical learning for the beginning student should not contain the same criteria as the evaluation tool for seniors. Exhibit 11–1 illustrates the use of the same critical objective for four nursing courses by increasing the complexity of the critical elements.

Appropriate Methods of Evaluation

The evaluation of clinical performance can be done by direct observation, videotape, written simulations, simulation laboratories, self-evaluations, and written assignments. Any of these methods can be used to assess the knowledge and/or performance of the student. Exclusive use of direct observation is time-consuming and often results in samples that are inadequate and not representative. See Suggested Readings for sources of in-depth discussion of evaluative techniques other than direct observation.

Infante addresses the use of the college laboratory as a creditable evaluative tool.[5] Many aspects of clinical performance could be evaluated much more effectively in the college learning laboratory than in the clinical area, but that would necessitate having competent clinical evaluators in the laboratory.

Here, as in the clinical setting, the student/teacher ratio should be low enough to permit learning and evaluation to occur. If the ratio is too high, validity of the evaluation may be sacrificed for speed. The clinical teacher in the college lab should attempt to simulate the clinical area by manipulating the environment to provide noise and distraction so common in agencies.

Formative and Summative Evaluations

Two types of evaluation that are very suitable for clinical instruction are formative and summative evaluations. *Formative evaluations* are "the assessments that are made during the teaching-learning process to monitor the progress of students and provide feedback to students."[6] *Summative evaluation,* on the other hand, is the final assessment of student achievement after a designated period

Exhibit 11–1 Leveling of Critical Elements for One Critical Objective

Critical Elements for Nursing 101

III. COMMUNICATION

Utilizes effective communication skills.

	Mid. S | U	Fin. S | U	Comments
• Develops an appropriate relationship with client.			
• Supports the concepts of "upright posture."			
• Maintains eye contact.			
• Uses appropriate verbal communication.			
• Responds appropriately to client's communications.			
• Displays a nonjudgmental attitude during nurse-client interactions.			
• Uses appropriate nonverbal communication.			
• Listens to the client.			
• Informs the instructor of client status.			
• Keeps instructor apprised of learning progress.			
• Writes appropriate nurse's notes.			
• Reports to appropriate persons.			

Critical Elements for Nursing 102

III. COMMUNICATION

Utilizes effective communication skills.

	Mid. S | U	Fin. S | U	Comments
• Develops effective relationships.			
• Uses appropriate verbal and nonverbal communication.			
• Uses appropriate terminology when communicating with others.			

Exhibit 11–1 continued

	Mid.		Fin.		Comments
	S	U	S	U	
• Communciates appropriately with all age groups.					
• Demonstrates appropriate interpersonal relationships with others.					
• Communicates to the client on the level of the learner.					
• Writes pertinent nurse's notes.					
• Writes concise nurse's notes.					
• Uses appropriate terminology in charting.					
• Reports discrepancies in health care to appropriate persons.					

Critical Elements for Nursing 201

III. COMMUNICATION

Utilizes therapeutic communication with client and family throughout the health-illness continuum.

	S	U	Comments
• Develops a therapeutic relationship.			
• Utilizes appropriate attending skills.			
• Communicates effectively with all age groups.			
• Demonstrates appropriate interpersonal relationships with others.			
• Verbalizes own attitudes, values, and feelings with regard to health care situations.			
• Informs the instructors of changes in client status.			

Critical Elements for Nursing 202 (Terminal Objective)

III. COMMUNICATION

Utilizes therapeutic communication with the client and family to promote optimum well-being.

	Mid.		Fin.		Comments
	S	U	S	U	
• Develops a therapeutic relationship.					
• Utilizes appropriate attending skills.					

Exhibit 11–1 continued

	Mid.		Fin.		
	S	U	S	U	Comments
• Uses effective verbal and nonverbal communication.					
• Uses appropriate terminology when communicating with others.					
• Communicates effectively with all age groups.					
• Demonstrates appropriate interpersonal relationships with others.					
• Verbalizes own attitudes, values, and feelings with regard to health care situations.					
• Informs the instructor and team leader of changes in client status.					
• Keeps the instructor apprised of learning progress.					
• Records client information appropriately.					

of time, as the end of a course or a program. Information gathered during formative evaluations may or may not be used in the summative evaluation of a student. Whereas formative evaluations examine incidents and events related to student learning, summative evaluations survey the patterns of behavior noted in a group of events and incidents.

The educator must emphasize the formative evaluation as a means of coaching the learner to identify and overcome weaknesses. Each incident is reviewed to identify areas of achievement and areas that need improvement. The learner should cite these weak and strong areas in the weekly log or self-evaluation.

The midterm conference may be used as a summative evaluation. The educator would at this time summarize all the events of the past semester and identify any pattern in behavior or clinical performance. The summative evaluation is used at the midterm when a grade is desired by the program or when specific objectives must be met at certain levels. Using the summative evaluation at midterm gives students concrete information about their standing in the educational program. If a student's performance has been unsatisfactory during the first half of a semester, midterm evaluation is a chance to warn the student of impending failure. Both individuals should sign evaluation forms as a routine practice. Signatures by both parties prevent the learner from protesting in the future "I never was told . . ."

Multifaculty Input

If in the evaluation period, more than one instructor is evaluating a student, the evaluation tool can be designed for multiple faculty input. It would be more prudent for a faculty member who supervises a student for only a week or two to add to the overall evaluation than to attempt to summarize incidents. These additions would be formative evaluations.

If at the conclusion of the teaching-learning process a final grade is assigned, it is advised that the period be divided in half with a designated midterm point. The midterm evaluation would provide students with an evaluation of their performance and with recommendations. Students should be given the opportunity to examine their performance and be aware of possible problem areas. It is not advised that the midterm evaluation be waived even when the evaluation period is short, e.g., two to four weeks.

In situations where an instructor has the students for four weeks, the grade assigned at the conclusion could reflect a midterm grade. At the end of the evaluation period, two instructors can then collaborate on the final grade. Exhibit 11–2 is an example of an evaluation tool that several instructors can utilize.

Anecdotal/Progress Records and Conferences

The importance of good and complete recordkeeping for evaluation cannot be overstated. This is not usually evident until a situation arises that necessitates reference to previous records. Without written records, by that time, usually at the end of the evaluation period, it is often too late to reconstruct past events. Time can dull the memory about specifics. Moreover, a conflict between the learner and the evaluator has already formed, partially perhaps because the learner was not kept aware of his or her progress or lack of progress.

The records to keep are anecdotal records, evaluations (midterm and final), and counseling conferences.

Anecdotal records or progress notes (see Exhibit 11–3) are objective records of incidents that support or refute student progress. These notations should be recorded as soon as possible after the incident. Since clinical days are often very busy, the educator may find taping anecdotes practical. Dictating the incidents while driving home from the hospital or clinic can save a great deal of time. The notes can be transcribed at a later time by a secretary or the educator.

Another way for recording anecdotal notes is to use the assignment sheets. The educator retains a carbon copy of each assignment sheet and uses the back to record incidents. This information about the client and specific interventions will

Exhibit 11-2 Evaluation Tool Providing for Multifaculty Input

	Evaluation Period #1						Evaluation Period #2						Evaluation Period #3						Anecdotal Incidents
	Strong	Average	Weak	Unsatisfactory	Unable to Evaluate		Strong	Average	Weak	Unsatisfactory	Unable to Evaluate		Strong	Average	Weak	Unsatisfactory	Unable to Evaluate		
6. Administers prescribed medications:																			
a. Safely																			
b. Demonstrates knowledge of classification, action, usage of those medications being administered.																			
c. Identifies factor(s) in client's status that is (are) affected by medications being delivered.																			
d. Demonstrates skill in making nursing judgments during the medication administration process.																			
e. Assesses proper procedure, scheduled time of administration, etc., of the various medications.																			
f. Demonstrates the ability to organize the administration of medications according to established priority of needs.																			
g. Demonstrates the ability to administer medications within prevailing ethical and legal standards of care.																			
h. To a group of 8-10 clients.																			

Signature Instructor

Signature Student

Date

Exhibit 11–3 Anecdotal Record Form

STUDENT _____	DATE _____
COURSE _____	FACULTY _____
SATISFACTORY	UNSATISFACTORY
DATE BEHAVIORS	DATE BEHAVIORS

help to recall incidents for discussion by the learner and the educator during counseling sessions.

The faculty can also design a progress note form organized on the critical clinical objectives with spaces to record comments and specific incidents. Exhibit 11–2 illustrates such a record.

Some educators believe that indicating to a learner that his or her performance is unsatisfactory early in the process causes the learner's anxiety to increase and creates more unsatisfactory performance. As mentioned previously, however, the evaluator should be involved in coaching instead of failing, and this information will assist the student in the learning process. The learner should be told of specific behaviors that need improvement.

Counseling conferences can be initiated by the instructor or the learner. The tone of a counseling session will depend greatly upon the personality of the counselor. If successful counseling is to take place, the educator-counselor must exhibit tolerance, sensitivity, and understanding. Individuals who seek assistance from a counselor must feel free to say anything without the threat of reprimand, disapproval, or punishment. An atmosphere of tolerance will encourage honesty and openness without fear of retaliation. Sensitivity and caring are essential qualities in a counseling session in order for a trusting relationship to develop. Sensitivity means that the counselor perceives, responds, and communicates the feelings and emotional tones of the person receiving counseling. The counselor must react to the moods of the other and understand that certain conflicts are causing the anxieties and frustrations. All this must be conveyed to the novice in an atmosphere of warmth and compassion.

Understanding means that the counselor realizes the novice's situation. Never having had the exact same experience under identical conditions, a counselor should still be able intellectually and emotionally to grasp what is being said. An accepting attitude means that the counselor is willing to permit others to be themselves. The individual's worth and dignity and right to make decisions must be acknowledged.

Grievance Procedures

A mechanism by which a student can formally disagree with an instructor's decision should be clearly outlined in the policy and student handbook. It is imperative that this procedure and the grievance committee that is a part of it be viewed as fair by both faculty and students. Grievance procedures are also discussed in Chapter 3.

In establishing a grievance procedure, the following elements should be addressed:

1. Confidentiality of the process
2. Committee membership (faculty, students)
3. Procedure
   - formal notification of grievance to committee after attempts for resolution have failed at the instructor, coordinator, and administrator level
   - deadline for notification, e.g., 30 days after receiving the official decision
4. Hearing
   - documents
   - witnesses
   - advisers
   - procedure for recording hearing (written, taped)

The grievance procedure is established to consider the reversal of a faculty decision. The two grounds for reversal of a clinical grade are proven faculty bias or proof that the instructor did not adhere to previously announced standards.

To prove bias, the student must present incidents where the instructor treated him or her differently (unfairly) from other students. At the hearing, the student will be asked to present evidence of bias. The committee should be cautioned not to attempt to establish why bias is present, only if it is present.

Prior to the hearing, both parties will be asked to submit all documents that relate to the grievance to the committee. Both parties will receive copies of the other's documents. Committee members may expedite the hearing if they review the documents prior to that day.

The chairperson conducts the hearing, providing each party and committee members with opportunities to relate and respond to presented information. After the committee has deliberated, the decision is forwarded in writing to all parties.

In the event that the decision is in favor of the student, it would be advisable that the student be given another opportunity to be evaluated by another faculty member, rather than just reversing the decision. Even though a faculty member used poor judgment, the committee cannot be assured that the student should be arbitrarily passed.

In order for the committee to be viewed as legitimate and fair, its decisions should be considered final except in a university setting where decisions at the college level can be appealed at the university level. If a dean or chairperson can reverse a grievance committee decision, the credibility of the committee or process is jeopardized.

THE FAILING OR UNSATISFACTORY STUDENT

"Clinical teaching of nursing is usually an exciting, rewarding experience for students and educators, for it is in the clinical setting that the art and science of nursing becomes most visible."[7] The assignment of a failing clinical grade to a student disrupts the entire experience and debilitates those involved. The prospect of failing a nursing course presents a different situation from failing a non-nursing course. Nursing students are often dedicated to becoming nurses, and many have a history of always having wanted to be a nurse. To such students failing means shattered dreams and plummeting self-esteem. Since the student may be unable to repeat the course until the next year, a financial burden may ensue.

The best planning does not prevent clinical failures but certain strategies can help to reduce the anger, hostility, guilt, and emotional distancing for the student and educator. In addition to the strategies discussed previously in this chapter, the following can assist in providing constructive interactions for all involved:

- coaching
- counseling sessions
- weekly student self-evaluations
- clinical probation
- faculty support

Coaching

Because the prospect of failing is a real threat to the student's self-esteem, the student may respond to it with guilt, anger, or hostility. In an attempt to reduce the intensity of these responses, the educator strives to maintain a coaching role to assist the student in focusing on selected incidents. The positive aspects of the student's performance must also be cited to enhance self-esteem. If the faculty member cannot identify any positive aspects in the student, it would be more prudent for another faculty member to evaluate the student.[8]

If a student refuses to agree with the evaluations, the educator may respond by trying to gather more data to justify the decision. Unfortunately, time must be spent gathering evidence rather than coaching the student to improve. The educator bombards the student with minor imperfections: a practice that usually creates more hostility and resentment. The instructor should minimize defending a decision and focus instead on significant behaviors.

Counseling Sessions

Maintaining an open dialogue is difficult, especially in the presence of hostility. Asking the student what she or he is most concerned about may identify for the educator areas that the student can be assisted with, for example, parents, finances, career goals. Faculty should be cautioned against telling a student that he or she should not be a nurse. Instead, it is best to focus on the fact that the student has not achieved satisfactory performance of clinical objectives. Career counseling should not be done by the instructor but rather by the program administrator or counselor.

Failing students may be unable to effectively deal with their families. Perhaps nursing was a career goal of the parents and not the student. The student may be relieved that the ordeal is over. In such cases the educator may offer to meet with the family to explain the situation. Several issues may be relevant:

- Did the family know the student was doing poorly at midterm?
- Does the family understand the complex nature of professional nursing or are nurses seen only as caring, nurturing individuals?
- Does the family understand that the curriculum is structured with increasing complexity?
- Does the family believe that anyone who wants to be a nurse can?
- Does the family know of the positive aspects of the student and what future options are available?

Weekly Student Self-Evaluation

Besides allowing learners to review their clinical behavior and place a value judgment on their performance, the weekly log gives the educator an idea of the learner's perception of his or her individual progress. It encourages the learner to recognize both behavior that improved and behavior in need of improvement. When the learner's log shows a perception of performance different from the instructor's, a conference should be scheduled to explore the disparity.

Clinical Probation

The clinical evaluation tool usually consists of two grade categories—unsatisfactory or satisfactory. Too often faculty are reluctant to assign a failing grade at midterm. To clearly communicate to a student that unless certain performance behaviors are corrected, they will fail, another category can be added at midterm. The category, clinical probation, allows the instructor to evaluate more behaviors before making a final decision and also alerts the student.

Unless an extreme situation occurs, students who are not placed on clinical probation at midterm are not failed, for if the deficiencies were not identified by midterm, perhaps the student was not given ample opportunity to pass. Exhibit 11–4 illustrates a form that is completed by the instructor and forwarded to the student at midterm.

A clinical probation must be removed at the end of the clinical course by a satisfactory or passing grade. A policy could also be established that if a student is placed on clinical probation more than once, termination is indicated.

Clinical probation

- provides the student and family with a clear indication that clinical performance is questionable
- supplies subsequent faculty with more data to support their decisions

---

Exhibit 11–4 Clinical Probation Form

STUDENT

COURSE

DATE

Clinical performance behaviors that need to be improved:

Additional comments, if indicated:

Student's comments (optional):

_____signature (instructor)
_____signature (student)
This signature does not mean I agree or disagree, only that I have read this form.

- offers faculty who usually do not fail students an opportunity to document borderline students
- represents a respectable structure for passing on information about a student's performance to other instructors

Faculty Support

Problems may occur when other faculty members do not agree with the educator's decision. At faculty meetings, instructors should indicate early in the semester the students who are having some difficulty. Faculty will then be prepared for the decision to fail the student if it is made.

Sometimes it is helpful for two educators to visit the clinical area to observe a borderline or failing student. Although this is often not feasible, it may be helpful to an inexperienced educator.

Failing a student clinically is an emotionally disturbing experience, and faculty need the support of their colleagues. If certain faculty acquire the reputation of "failing instructors," this may be because other faculty never assign failing grades. We must cease viewing the faculty person who fails students as cruel and uncaring, but instead begin to see this action as a higher form of caring—responsibility and accountability to the student, the client, and the profession.

FACULTY EVALUATION

The discussion of faculty evaluations will be restricted to the evaluation of clinical faculty by the learner. Some areas that can be evaluated are as follows:

- Availability (on and off the clinical sites)
- Clinical competency
- Announced standards
- Consistency

The practice of allowing the learner to evaluate faculty anonymously should be questioned. The learner should have to substantiate his or her evaluations just as the educator must. Criticism takes a different and often a more constructive form when the author must identify himself or herself.

The educator should meet with the learner to review the evaluation. The educator should ask for clarification if needed but must be receptive. If the learner is expected to be receptive to criticism, then the educator must be a role model.

The purpose of this evaluation is for the learner to help the educator to find which teaching techniques need improvement. The learner should also identify techniques that are especially beneficial.

The learner needs help in developing evaluating skills. Practicing nurses may be involved in peer evaluations, and if they become first-line managers or educators, evaluations will be mandatory. The learner can be helped to appreciate the evaluation process and to identify techniques to create a constructive process.

The process of evaluation can provide the educator and the learner with the feedback to alter or to encourage selected performances. A well-planned process can influence mutual satisfaction and acceptance by both parties. A caring, prudent educator can reduce or eliminate the frustration and anger that often accompany evaluations.

SUMMARY

The teaching of nursing can be a creative, rewarding experience or a frustrating, debilitating one. The outcome depends on how carefully planned the learning experiences are. The nurse educator strives to provide productive, humanistic experiences for the learner. For only in an environment of mutual respect and freedom can a learner evolve into a dynamic, empathetic professional advocate of clients.

NOTES

1. Patricia Benner and Judith Wrubel, "Skill Clinical Knowledge: The Value of Perceptual Awareness." *Part I American Journal of Nursing* 82 (May 1982): 11.

2. Ibid., p. 12.

3. Janice M. Stecchi, Sheryd J. Woltman, et al. "Comprehensive Approach to Clinical Evaluation: One Teaching Teams's Solution to Clinical Evaluation of Students in Multiple Settings." *Journal of Nursing Education* 22 (January 1983): 38.

4. Ibid., p. 38.

5. Lynda Juall Carpenito, "The Failing or Unsatisfactory Student." *Nurse Educator* 8 (Winter 1983): 32.

6. Ibid., p. 32.

7. Ibid., p. 32.

8. Ibid., p. 33.

SUGGESTED READINGS

Bernabei, Raymond, and Sam Leles. *Behavioral Objectives in Curriculum and Evaluation.* Dubuque, Iowa: Kendall/Hunt, 1970.

Capobianco, Anna T. "The Development of a System for Evaluation." National League for Nursing Pub. 23-1775, 1979.

Carpenito, Lynda Juall. "The Failing or Unsatisfactory Student." *Nurse Educator* 8, no. 4 (Winter 1983): 32–33.

Frisbee, David A. "Evaluating Student Achievement." National League for Nursing Pub. 23-1766, 1979.

Haar, L.P., and J.R. Hicks. "Performance Appraisal: Derivation of Effective Assessment Tools." *The Journal of Nursing Administration* 76, no. 9 (September 1976): 20–29.

Infante, Mary Sue. *The Clinical Laboratory in Nursing Education*. New York: John Wiley, 1975.

Kelly, Ruth L. "Evaluation Is More Than a Measurement." *American Journal of Nursing* 73, no. 1 (January 1973): 114–116.

MacKinnon, Harold, and Lillian Erikson. "C.A.R.E.—A Four Track Professional Nurse Classification and Performance Evaluation System." *The Journal of Nursing Administration* (April 1977): 42–44.

Morgan, B., et al. "Evaluating Clinical Proficiency." *Nursing Outlook* 27 (August 1979): 540–544.

Morgan, Margaret, and David Irby. *Evaluating Clinical Competence in the Health Professions*. St. Louis: C.V. Mosby, 1978.

Reilly, Dorothy E. *Behavioral Objectives in Nursing: Evaluation of Learner Attainment*. New York: Appleton-Century-Crofts, 1975.

Stainton, M. Colleen. "A Format for Recording the Clinical Performance of Nursing Students." *Journal of Nursing Education* 22, no. 3 (March 1983): 114–116.

Stecchi, Janice, et al. "Comprehensive Approach to Clinical Evaluation: One Teaching's Team's Solution to Clinical Evaluation of Students in Multiple Settings." *Journal of Nursing Education* 22, no. 1 (January 1983): 38–46.

Stevens, Barbara J. "Performance Appraisal: What the Nurse Executive Expects from It." *The Journal of Nursing Administration* 76, no. 10 (October 1976): 26–31.

Voight, J.W. "Assessing Clinical Performance: A Model for Competency." *Journal of Nursing Education* 18 (April 1979): 30–33.

Wakim, Judith H. "A Workable In-Depth Curriculum Evaluation Plan." *Nurse Educator* 8, no. 3 (Autumn 1983): 24–32.

Woolley, Alma. "The Long and Tortured History of Clinical Evaluation." *Nursing Outlook* 25, no. 5 (May 1977): 303–315.

Appendix 11–A

Clinical Evaluation Based on Critical Elements

Clarion University
Division of Nursing
Associate Degree Nursing Program

Evaluation of Clinical Progress

Nursing 202

Student _____   Dates of Experience _____

Professor _____   _____

_____   Evaluation: Self _____ Instructor _____

Date of Conference _____   Mid-term _____ Final _____
_____   (red)   (blue)

Grade _____   S = Satisfactory Performance
_____   U = Unsatisfactory Performance

*Critical Elements:

	Mid.		Fin.	
	S	U	S	U
I. Maintains the physical safety of the client.				

	Mid.		Fin.	
	S	U	S	U
II. Utilizes the nursing process.				

	Mid.		Fin.	
	S	U	S	U
III. Communicates appropriately.				

240

	Mid.		Fin.	
	S	U	S	U
IV. Demonstrates accountability and responsibility.				

*All critical elements must be met in order to pass the course.

I. TECHNICAL SKILLS

A. Demonstrates proficiency in providing nursing intervention to the client and family through-out the health-illness continuum.

	Mid.		Fin.		Comments
	S	U	S	U	
1. Maintains client safety.					
2. Carries out the prescribed nursing and medical care correctly.					
3. Identifies inconsistencies in the prescribed nursing and medical regimens.					
4. Administers treatments safely.					
5. Administers medications safely.					
6. Demonstrates competency in I.V. therapy.					

II. NURSING PROCESS

A. Utilizes the nursing process to formulate a comprehensive plan of care with the client and family.

	Mid.		Fin.		Comments
	S	U	S	U	
1. Makes valid assessments.					
2. Validates information with appropriate sources.					
3. Makes appropriate nursing diagnoses based upon priorities of client needs.					
4. Establishes realistic long-term and short-term goals with the client and family.					
5. Develops a comprehensive nursing care plan with client and family.					
6. Makes appropriate judgments concerning client care.					

	Mid. S | U	Fin. S | U	Comments
7. Plans with the client the activities of daily living.			
8. Makes valid additions to nursing unit's care plans.			
9. Implements the nursing care plan according to priority of needs.			
10. Evaluates the effectiveness of nursing interventions.			
11. Revises the nursing care plan on a continuing basis.			
12. Asks for assistance from appropriate persons.			
13. Delegates non-nursing activities effectively.			

B. Incorporates health teaching in the care of the client and family throughout their life processes.

	Mid. S | U	Fin. S | U	Comments
1. Develops an accurate and individualized health teaching plan according to client needs.			
2. Utilizes the principles of the teaching-learning process in implementing the health teaching plan.			
3. Evaluates the effectiveness of the teaching.			
4. Evaluates the degree of client comprehension and the likelihood of his compliance.			

III. COMMUNICATION

A. Utilizes therapeutic communication with the client and family to promote opimum well-being.

	Mid. S | U	Fin. S | U	Comments
1. Develops a therapeutic relationship.			
2. Utilizes appropriate attending skills.			
3. Uses effective verbal and nonverbal communication.			

	Mid.		Fin.		
	S	U	S	U	Comments
4. Uses appropriate terminology when communicating with others.					
5. Communicates effectively with all age groups.					
6. Demonstrates appropriate interpersonal relationships with others.					
7. Verbalizes own attitudes, values and feelings with regard to health care situations.					
8. Informs the instructor and team leader of changes in client status.					
9. Keeps the instructor apprised of learning progress.					
10. Records client information appropriately.					

IV. RESPONSIBILITY AND ACCOUNTABILITY

A. Demonstrates responsibility and accountability for self-direction and self-evaluation.

	Mid.		Fin.		
	S	U	S	U	Comments
1. Takes the initiative in the learning process.					
2. Seeks opportunities for learning.					
3. Incorporates appropriate suggestions into learning experiences.					
4. Demonstrates evidence of preparation for clinical experience.					
5. Utilizes a variety of resources in preparations for clinical experience.					
6. Contributes appropriately to conferences.					
7. Evaluates realistically own performance including strengths and weaknesses.					
8. Displays assertive behavior.					

B. Demonstrates responsibility and accountability for nursing care.

	Mid.		Fin.		
	S	U	S	U	Comments
1. Demonstrates self-confidence.					
2. Assumes responsibility for own actions.					

	Mid.		Fin.		Comments
	S	U	S	U	
3. Demonstrates responsibility to the client and family.					
4. Demonstrates responsibility and accountability for comprehensive client care.					

Performs at expected levels of competency: (Mid)   Passing _____   Failing _____
                                              (Final) Passing _____   Failing _____

Instructor's Comment:

Instructor's signature:

(Mid) _____
                                                    Date

(Final) _____
                                                    Date

Student's Comment:

Student's signature:

(Mid) _____
                                                    Date

(Final) _____
                                                    Date

This signature does not mean I agree or disagree, only that I have read this evaluation.

Source: Reprinted with permission of Clarion University of Pennsylvania, Division of Nursing.

Index